WORKBOOK
FOR
Essentials of Human Diseases and Conditions

fourth edition

Margaret Schell Frazier, RN, CMA, BS
Retired
Former Chair, Health and Human Services Division
Program Chair, Medical Assisting Program
Ivy Tech State College, Northeast
Fort Wayne, Indiana

Jeanette Wist Drzymkowski, RN, BS
Formerly
Associate Faculty
Ivy Tech State College, Northeast
Fort Wayne, Indiana

SAUNDERS

ELSEVIER

SAUNDERS
ELSEVIER

11830 Westline Industrial Drive
St. Louis, Missouri 63146

Workbook for
ESSENTIALS OF HUMAN DISEASES AND CONDITIONS   ISBN-13: 978-1-4160-4715-5

Notice
Knowledge and best practice in this field are constantly changing. As new research and experience broaden our knowledge, changes in practice, treatment and drug therapy may become necessary or appropriate. Readers are advised to check the most current information provided (i) on procedures featured or (ii) by the manufacturer of each product to be administered, to verify the recommended dose or formula, the method and duration of administration, and contraindications. It is the responsibility of the practitioner, relying on their own experience and knowledge of the patient, to make diagnoses, to determine dosages and the best treatment for each individual patient, and to take all appropriate safety precautions. To the fullest extent of the law, neither the Publisher nor the Author assumes any liability for any injury and/or damage to persons or property arising out of or related to any use of the material contained in this book.
The Publisher

Previous editions copyrighted 2004, 2000, 1996

ISBN-13: 978-1-4160-4715-5

Executive Editor: Susan Cole
Developmental Editor: Celeste Clingan
Publishing Services Manager: Pat Joiner-Myers
Project Manager: David Stein
Design Direction: Teresa McBryan

Printed in United States

Working together to grow
libraries in developing countries
www.elsevier.com | www.bookaid.org | www.sabre.org

ELSEVIER   BOOK AID International   Sabre Foundation

Last digit is the print number: 9 8 7 6 5 4

Developing an understanding to disease processes is an exciting and fascinating facet of the health care provider's education. Considering that disease conditions are universally experienced, most of us have a natural curiosity about them; however, it is essential that we as health care providers also are cognizant of the many components of disease. The study of current medical information on the more common clinical disorders encountered in the health care field presents a challenge to any student.

Essentials of Human Diseases and Conditions, fourth edition, attempts to condense and simplify current medical information on the more common clinical disorders encountered in the health field and physician's office. This companion workbook is intended to present an orderly and concise review of information and to assist you in investigating diseases of the human body. The authors of this workbook, both medical-assisting educators and RNs, recognize how essential it is for you to have an organized means of reinforcing and reviewing information presented in the text and during class sessions. It is our goal to provide a tool that will bolster the educational experience as you study pathophysiology, as well as one that will help you approach learning the basics of the human pathologic condition.

Students have previously expressed their desire to have a workbook or study guide to help with studying notes and preparing for examinations. This workbook is a means to review pertinent information, making it more likely that you will remember diseases along with their signs, symptoms, and treatments.

This workbook has been planned to follow the textbook chapters in an orderly fashion. Each chapter of the workbook follows the body systems and presents the review material in the following order:
- Word Definitions
- Glossary Terms
- Short Answer
- Fill in the Blanks
- Anatomic Structures
- Patient Screening
- Patient Teaching
- Pharmacology Questions
- Essay Questions
- Certification Examination Review (Multiple Choice)

WORD DEFINITIONS

The sections titled Word Definitions list essential words to help you develop and understand disease entities. The use of a medical dictionary or medical terminology book may be necessary to arrive at the correct meaning of each word as it is used in the textbook.

GLOSSARY TERMS

Glossary terms are boldfaced and/or italicized in each chapter and presented in the glossary section in the back of the textbook. It is suggested that you attempt to recall the information presented in class lectures and then confirm the definition with the textbook glossary.

SHORT ANSWER

Short-answer questions are included in each chapter as a method of providing you with a means of recall. These questions address pertinent facts of selected diseases discussed in the chapter.

FILL IN THE BLANKS

Fill-in-the-blank questions provide an opportunity for you to apply one-word or short answers, again to help reinforce and review the information presented. Answers are provided in Word Lists for rapid recognition.

ANATOMIC STRUCTURES

Illustrations of anatomic structures and processes are included for labeling. Knowledge of anatomy is crucial to understanding the concepts of disease processes. These labeling exercises are intended to enhance learning.

PATIENT SCREENING

Selected patient-screening scenarios are presented to enable you to relate how you would handle telephone calls to the medical office. For these exercises, you should apply the following general guidelines for patient screening in combination with critical thinking skills to formulate a typical screening response. Five typical phone calls are presented per chapter.

GUIDELINES FOR PATIENT-SCREENING EXERCISES

Typically, the medical assistant has the responsibility of screening telephone calls from patients requesting an appointment or reporting treatment progress or lack of progress. The medical assistant is often the initial contact for the patient or patient's family, and critical thinking and a prompt response are required. Many offices have established guidelines regarding the extent of assessment that can be made over the telephone in compliance with state practice acts. It is essential that office staff be aware of and follow office guidelines. Additionally, the medical assistant who is answering the phone may have a list of questions that he or she is expected to ask along with suggestions for appropriate responses regarding appointments or acceptable referrals. Important guidelines for life-threatening situations are listed in the textbook and in this workbook.

It is recommended that you review the information in the text regarding patient screening. The guidelines listed are not intended for diagnosing a caller's medical condition or for providing curative advice. These exercises offer general clues to enable you to recognize the urgency for an appointment, to identify individuals reporting an emergency, and to discern the kind of calls that require referral to the physician for response. These exercises are not intended to focus on the skill of medical triage, which state practice acts generally reserve for certain licensed professionals. When a patient calls, careful listening is essential because the caller often relays information that will help the medical assistant to decide the appropriate action required. Ideally, the outcome of telephone communication between caller and screener will benefit the patient and avoid potential medical and legal problems. The importance of sensitivity to human suffering, strict confidentiality, and a keen awareness of the priority of meeting the needs of patients are necessary skills of the telephone screener and cannot be overstated. The medical assistant must always keep in mind the following important facts:

- Only physicians and nurse practitioners may diagnose disease and prescribe medications.
- Established office protocol must always be followed during the screening process.
- All calls and referrals must be documented according to office policy.

The following serious and life-threatening conditions require immediate assessment and intervention:

- Sudden onset of unexplained shortness of breath
- Crushing pain across the center of the chest
- Difficult breathing occurring suddenly and rapidly worsening, often in the middle of the night
- Vomiting bright red or very dark coffee-grounds–appearing blood
- Sudden onset of weakness and unsteadiness or severe dizziness
- Sudden loss of consciousness or paralysis
- Flashes of light in field of vision
- Sudden and progressively worsening abdominal, flank, or pelvic pain
- Sudden onset of blurred vision accompanied by severe throbbing in the eye

- Children and other individuals with a history of asthma and sudden onset of difficulty breathing

Additional symptoms requiring prompt assessment include but are not limited to:

- Sudden or recent onset of unexplained bleeding including blood in urine, stool, or emesis
- Coughing or spitting up of blood
- Unusual and unexplained or heavy vaginal bleeding
- Elevated body temperature of sudden onset or for a prolonged period
- Continued abdominal, back, or pelvic pain
- Sudden onset of headache-type pain
- Children with elevated temperatures or continued vomiting
- Infants with sudden onset of projectile vomiting

It is essential to document all calls according to office policy and to notify the physician in an emergency situation.

PATIENT TEACHING

Selected patient-teaching scenarios are included to enable you to convey how you would handle patient-teaching opportunities in the medical office. For these exercises, you should apply the following general guidelines for patient teaching.

GUIDELINES FOR PATIENT-TEACHING EXERCISES

The patient-teaching exercises are intended to provide you with an opportunity to develop patient-teaching skills. The actual implementation of these skills is dependent on state practice acts and office policies. You have the responsibility to make yourself aware of your state's practice acts and office policy before attempting actual patient teaching. Once you have ascertained that patient teaching is within your scope of practice, you should check office policy for suggested protocol. Many offices have established guidelines for patient teaching, as well as printed materials to assist the health care professional in patient-teaching responsibilities.

- Most offices have patient instructions that are written on the encounter form at the end of the physician's contact with the patient.
- As the patient signs out or before he or she leaves the examination room, the medical assistant reviews these instructions with the patient.
- Often the scheduling of a return visit is the only instruction the physician may write.

Other identified instructions may be the scheduling of additional testing or the inclusion of information about diets or prescribed medications. Although these instructions are a form of patient teaching, reinforcing patient instructions and obtaining patient feedback that confirms his or her understanding of the instructional material are usually considered essential responsibilities for any health care provider.

You are encouraged to review general principles of patient teaching as provided in the text.

- It is important to remember that the patient is a partner in health care and that patient teaching, as an ongoing process, requires interaction with the patient and his or her family or caregiver.
- Presenting the material to the patient must be done at the patient's level of understanding.

As you approach each patient-teaching experience, you should have a goal in mind. Usually patients express goals for a recovery or improvement in their health situation during the intake assessment procedure. Encouraging input from the patient and family or caregiver in setting goals and delegating responsibility for suggested procedures or activities are in the best interest of the patient. The development of a trusting relationship and effective communication help because individuals are encouraged to assume responsibility for their health and recovery.

The patient-teaching scenarios provided are possible patient-teaching opportunities for the health care professional. The scenarios are presented for every chapter except Chapter 1. You should describe how you would approach the appropriate teaching activity for each situation. Certain patient-teaching opportunities could be duplicated because many teaching concepts are generalized for similar conditions. Once wound care has been explained, it is not necessary for you to repeat this type of instruction in a detailed manner in similar scenarios. Daily weights and requirements for taking medications at the same time every day are examples of patient-teaching opportunities that apply to many patient-teaching situations. Handwashing reminders are an important factor to be mentioned in most teaching opportunities.

PHARMACOLOGY QUESTIONS

Pharmacology questions enhance and review pharmacology associated with treatment of diseases and conditions presented within each chapter. The exercises provide a means of identifying types of medication or therapies that are used to treat a patient in certain circumstances.

ESSAY QUESTIONS

One essay question is included for each chapter. These questions will provide you with an opportunity to discuss or explain in detail certain disease-related topics presented in the chapter.

CERTIFICATION EXAMINATION REVIEW

Multiple choice–style questions simulate the typical format found in the certification examination. These questions are incorporated to prepare students for what they will encounter in the certification examination.

It is our goal to furnish you with the optimal study instruments to achieve an understanding of the disease entities you may encounter in a physician's office. We wish you success in your endeavor.

Margaret Schell Frazier, RN, CMA, BS
Jeanette Wist Drzymkowski, RN, BS

Contents

CHAPTER 1

Mechanisms of Disease, Diagnosis, and Treatment

WORD DEFINITIONS

Define the following basic medical terms:

1. Adipose _____

2. Alopecia _____

3. Analgesic _____

4. Cognitive _____

5. Dysfunction _____

6. Ectopic _____

7. Endometrial _____

8. Genetic _____

9. Hematopoietic _____

10. Hypervitaminosis _____

11. Nosocomial _____

12. Palliative _____

13. Preoperatively _____

14. Reflexology _____

15. Systemic _____

16. Transcutaneous _____

17. Transient _____

18. Urticaria _____

19. Visceral _____

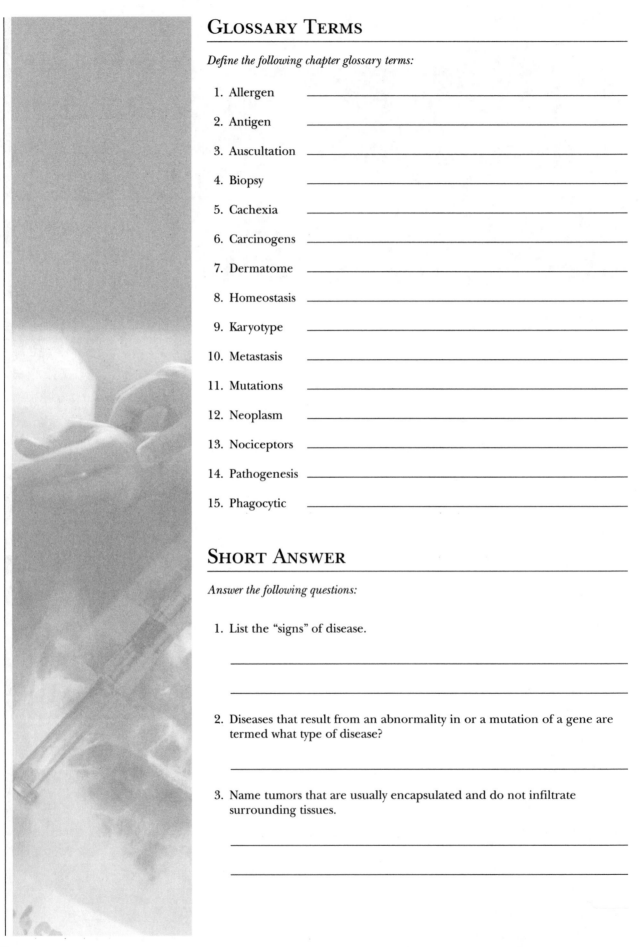

GLOSSARY TERMS

Define the following chapter glossary terms:

1. Allergen _____

2. Antigen _____

3. Auscultation _____

4. Biopsy _____

5. Cachexia _____

6. Carcinogens _____

7. Dermatome _____

8. Homeostasis _____

9. Karyotype _____

10. Metastasis _____

11. Mutations _____

12. Neoplasm _____

13. Nociceptors _____

14. Pathogenesis _____

15. Phagocytic _____

SHORT ANSWER

Answer the following questions:

1. List the "signs" of disease.

   _____

   _____

2. Diseases that result from an abnormality in or a mutation of a gene are termed what type of disease?

   _____

3. Name tumors that are usually encapsulated and do not infiltrate surrounding tissues.

   _____

   _____

4. Name tumors with invasive cells that multiply excessively and infiltrate other tissues that can represent a serious threat to the patient.

_____

_____

5. Identify the hormone that may be elevated when a patient has prostate cancer.

_____

6. Cite the statistics for the highest male and female new cancer cases and deaths in the United States, as estimated by the American Cancer Society.

_____

7. Any substance that causes an allergic response in a patient is called what?

_____

8. Identify the concept of care that is focused on family support and comfort during life threatening illness.

_____

9. What does MRSA refer to?

_____

10. What may be the cause of immunodeficiency disorders?

_____

11. What is the single greatest avoidable cause of death and disease?

_____

12. What information is valuable in helping a health care provider assess a patient's condition?

_____

13. What may the physician order to assist with the diagnosis of a patient?

_____

14. Scientists study stem cells to investigate their potential to repair damaged tissue in a field called

_____

_____

15. List some examples of predisposing factors related to lifestyle.

_____

_____

16. What are Staphylococcus and Streptococcus?

_____

17. Identify two environmental factors that may place a patient at increased risk for illnesses such as pulmonary disease and cancer.

_____

_____

18. Name the type of pain that is usually less severe and has duration of longer than 6 months. (Inflammatory conditions, such as arthritis and bursitis, are examples.)

_____

19. Name the classification of pain that usually has a sudden onset and is severe in intensity.

_____

20. Name the basic units of heredity that are a small part of a DNA molecule; they are located on chromosomes.

_____

21. Are there any genetic mutations compatible with life?

_____

22. What are the general treatment options for cancer?

_____

_____

23. Fever, headache, body aches, weakness, fatigue, loss of appetite, and delirium are all symptoms of what?

_____

24. What may be recommended when an individual is known to have a contagious disease that can be easily transmitted to others?

_____

25. Identify the simple precaution that is known to help prevent transmission of pathogens from one person to another, especially in hospital and outpatient medical settings.

_____

FILL IN THE BLANKS

Fill in the blanks with the correct terms. A word list has been provided.

1. Preventive health care emphasizes strategies for _____ a disease before it happens.

2. The X and Y chromosomes are known as _____ chromosomes.

3. Each person has _____ pairs of chromosomes. One chromosome from each pair is inherited from the _____ and one from the _____.

4. The cardinal signs of infection include _____, _____, _____, _____, _____, _____, and _____.

5. The _____ is a government agency responsible for publishing infectious disease reports in the United States after the diseases are reported to local health departments.

6. Tumors can be classified as either _____ or _____.

7. After evaluation, cancerous tissue is assigned a stage number ranging from I to IV, with stage _____ being an earlier stage tumor, which carries a better prognosis.

8. The _____ of cancer treatment is to eradicate every cancer cell in the body.

9. Chemotherapy involves the use of chemicals to eradicate cancer cells. The most common side effects are _____, _____, _____, _____, _____, _____, and _____.

10. Physical trauma is the most common cause of death in _____ and _____ _____.

11. A few examples of common allergens that are inhaled include _____, _____, and _____.

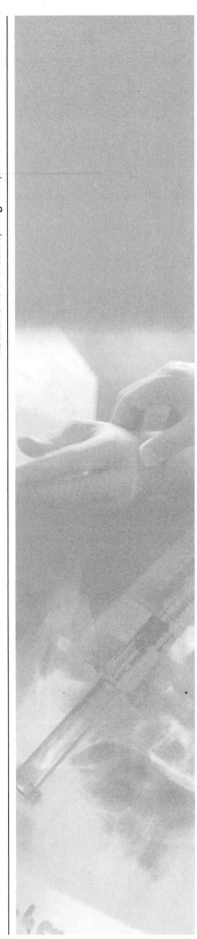

12. When a person experiences pain, it is a warning sign that

_____ _____ is occurring.

13. Cultural diversity is recognized in the _____ realm of

medical treatment because health care providers must meet the needs of

culturally diverse patients.

14. Reflexology directs its efforts to the massage of the _____

and _____.

15. Genetic counseling is helpful in predicting _____ of

_____ of a gene-linked disease in a family.

WORD LIST

I, 23, alopecia, anemia, anorexia, benign, bruising, Centers for Disease Control and Prevention (CDC), children, diarrhea, dust, enlarged lymph glands, father, feet, fever, fungi, goal, hands, heat, holistic, infertility, malignant, mold, mother, occurrence, pain, preventing, pus, redness, red streaks, risk, sex, swelling, tissue damage, vomiting, young adults

PHARMACOLOGY QUESTIONS

Circle the letter of the choice that best completes the statement or answers the question.

1. Medication issues for concern relating to the elderly include
   a. Adverse drug reactions.
   b. Substance abuse.
   c. Overmedication.
   d. All of the above.

2. Categories of infectious disease management medications include
   a. Antibacterials (antibiotics).
   b. Antifungal and antiviral medications.
   c. Anthelmintics.
   d. All of the above.

3. Medications prescribed for pain are termed
   a. Antipyretic.
   b. Analgesic.
   c. Antibiotic.
   d. Nutritional agent.

4. An epinephrine kit for self administration may be prescribed for an individual known to have severe
   a. Pain.
   b. Depression.
   c. Allergies.
   d. Diabetes.

ESSAY QUESTION

Write a response to the following question or statement. Use a separate sheet of paper if more space is needed.

Discuss the importance of recognizing cultural diversity in patients.

_____

_____

_____

_____

_____

_____

_____

_____

_____

_____

_____

_____

_____

CERTIFICATION EXAMINATION REVIEW

Circle the letter of the choice that best completes the statement or answers the question.

1. An abnormality in or mutation of a gene may produce which of the following?
   a. Inflammatory diseases
   b. Immunodeficiency disorders
   c. Genetic diseases
   d. None of the above

2. What types of tumors tend to metastasize and may spread to distant sites in the body?
   a. Malignant tumors
   b. Benign tumors
   c. Adipose tumors
   d. All of the above

3. Which of the following are included in the body's natural defense system against infection?
   a. Mechanical and chemical barriers
   b. Inflammatory response
   c. Immune response
   d. All of the above

4. Which of the following describe how a pathogen can cause disease?
   a. Intoxification
   b. Invasion and destruction of living tissue
   c. Infiltration of dead tissue
   d. Both a and b

5. Systemic manifestations of severe allergic responses include
   a. Arthralgia.
   b. Status asthmaticus.
   c. Anaphylaxis.
   d. All of the above.

6. The concept of medical care that focuses on the needs of the whole person—spiritual, cognitive, social, physical, and emotional—is the
   a. Holistic concept.
   b. Hospice concept.
   c. Osteopathy concept.
   d. None of the above

7. The concept of care that affirms life and neither hastens or postpones death is the
   a. Holistic concept.
   b. Hospice philosophy.
   c. Osteopathy concept.
   d. None of the above

8. Which of the following is responsible for stimulating the immune system to produce antibodies?
   a. Mutation
   b. Chromosome
   c. Antigen
   d. None of the above

9. A new tissue growth or a tumor is called a
   a. Mutation.
   b. Neoplasm.
   c. Biopsy.
   d. None of the above

10. Predisposing factors related to lifestyle include
    a. Gender.
    b. Age.
    c. Pollution of air and water.
    d. Smoking, poor nutrition, lack of exercise, risky sexual behavior.

11. Pain as described by the patient is
    a. Objective.
    b. Experienced the same in everyone.
    c. Subjective and individualized.
    d. Never referred to other regions of the body.

12. Patient education
    a. Helps improve patient and family coping.
    b. Is interactive.
    c. Is based on the patient's plan of care.
    d. All of the above

8

CHAPTER 2

Developmental, Congenital, and Childhood Diseases and Disorders

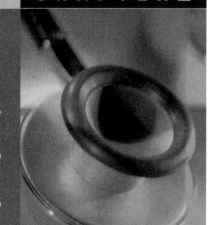

WORD DEFINITIONS

Define the following basic medical terms:

1. Adduction   _____

2. Apnea   _____

3. Arthritis   _____

4. Bursitis   _____

5. Congenital   _____

6. Hydrocephalus   _____

7. Hypovolemia   _____

8. Lethargy   _____

9. Myopia   _____

10. Nosocomial   _____

11. Palpable   _____

12. Posterior   _____

13. Postnatal   _____

14. Postpartum   _____

15. Tracheostomy   _____

16. Transdermal   _____

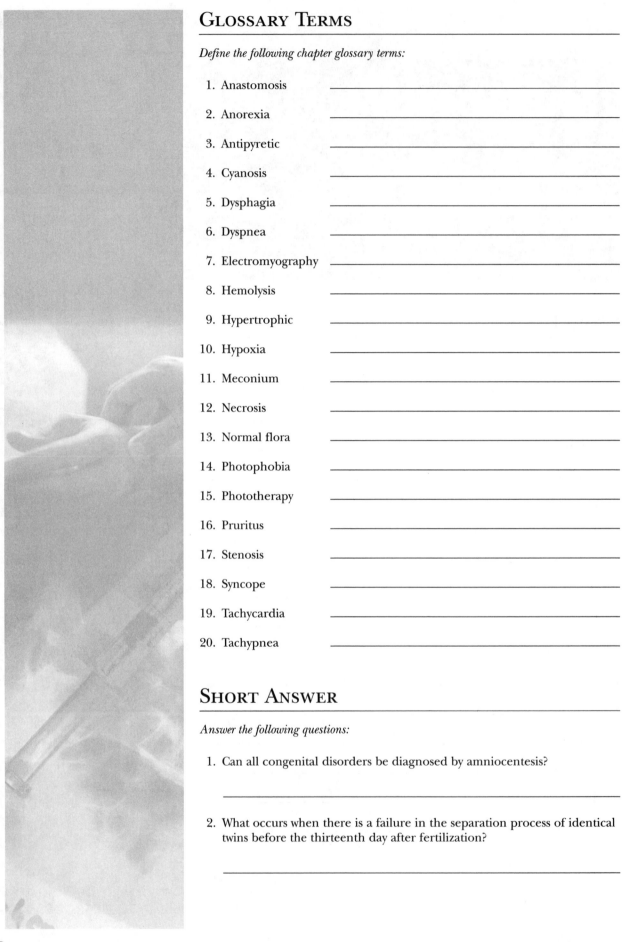

GLOSSARY TERMS

Define the following chapter glossary terms:

1. Anastomosis _____

2. Anorexia _____

3. Antipyretic _____

4. Cyanosis _____

5. Dysphagia _____

6. Dyspnea _____

7. Electromyography _____

8. Hemolysis _____

9. Hypertrophic _____

10. Hypoxia _____

11. Meconium _____

12. Necrosis _____

13. Normal flora _____

14. Photophobia _____

15. Phototherapy _____

16. Pruritus _____

17. Stenosis _____

18. Syncope _____

19. Tachycardia _____

20. Tachypnea _____

SHORT ANSWER

Answer the following questions:

1. Can all congenital disorders be diagnosed by amniocentesis?

   _____

2. What occurs when there is a failure in the separation process of identical twins before the thirteenth day after fertilization?

   _____

3. Is the condition of conjoined twins more prevalent in females or males?

   _____

4. What is the weight range for premature infants?

   _____

5. List three causes of prematurity.

   _____

6. Name an example of an abnormality that may be detected by examination of amniotic fluid.

   _____

7. What is another name for infant respiratory distress syndrome (IRDS)?

   _____

8. Explain how retinopathy of prematurity (retrolental fibroplasias) is diagnosed.

   _____

   _____

9. What is considered to be the most common crippling condition of children?

   _____

10. Is a patient with cerebral palsy always mentally retarded?

    _____

11. Identify the most serious form of spina bifida.

    _____

12. If a baby is born with anencephaly, what is the prognosis?

    _____

13. What are the two forms of Robinow syndrome?

    _____

14. Name the most common congenital cardiac disorder.

    _____

15. What color is the skin of a baby born with tetralogy of Fallot?

    _____

16. Cite the statistics for the occurrence of cleft abnormalities.

    _____

17. Name the most common kidney tumor of childhood.

_____

18. Is the cause of anemia the same in all cases?

_____

19. List examples of helminths that can live in the gastrointestinal (GI) tract.

_____

20. Klinefelter's syndrome and Turner's syndrome are both chromosomal disorders. Which one affects males, and which one affects females?

_____

21. The test for cystic fibrosis that measures the levels of sodium and chloride is called what?

_____

22. Identify the organism responsible for causing chickenpox.

_____

23. List a few precautions women can take to help decrease the risk of abnormal fetal development.

_____

24. Cite possible causes of nongenetic congenital abnormalities that may be present in a child.

_____

_____

25. List the three major types of cerebral palsy.

_____

_____

_____

26. Explain the goal of treatment for cerebral palsy.

_____

27. List the four abnormalities present in the heart of an infant who has tetralogy of Fallot.

_____

_____

_____

_____

28. What are some of the physical characteristics that a child with Down syndrome will exhibit?

_____

_____

29. Explain the treatment measures that may be used if clubfoot is present.

_____

_____

30. What treatment options are available to a baby born with patent ductus arteriosus (PDA)?

_____

_____

31. Define phimosis.

_____

32. List the symptoms associated with adenoid hyperplasia.

_____

33. What is the method of transmission for lead poisoning?

_____

FILL IN THE BLANKS

Fill in the blanks with the correct terms. A word list has been provided.

1. The diagnosis of congenital anomalies in a fetus can be accomplished by amniocentesis between the _____ and

   _____ week of pregnancy.

2. An infant with bronchopulmonary dysplasia (BPD) is very susceptible to respiratory infections, such as _____ and

   _____.

3. Muscular dystrophy is diagnosed by _____,

   _____, _____, and _____,

   _____, _____, _____.

4. The exact cause of spina bifida is unknown. However,

   _____ and _____ factors may play a role.

   In addition, a decrease in the amount of _____ and

   _____ may contribute to the occurrence.

5. Treatment for hydrocephalus usually includes placing a

_____ in the ventricular or subarachnoid spaces to drain

off the excessive cerebrospinal fluid (CSF).

6. An infant with cri du chat syndrome will exhibit an abnormally

_____ head, and if born alive, the infant will have a weak

_____, catlike cry.

7. Congenital _____ defects are developmental anomalies of

the heart or _____ of the heart.

8. An atrial septic defect that is large would cause pronounced symptoms of

_____, _____, and _____.

9. The prognosis for cleft lip and cleft palate is _____ with

surgical repair.

10. An infant with _____ _____ has episodes

of projectile vomiting after feedings. The onset of symptoms usually

begins within 2 to 3 weeks after birth.

11. Phenylketonuria is an inborn error in the metabolism of amino acids

that causes _____ _____ and

_____ _____ if not treated.

12. Diphtheria can be prevented by the administration of

_____ _____ to produce active immunity.

13. The causative agent of mumps is an _____ virus, which is

spread by _____ nuclei from the respiratory tract.

14. The drug of choice to treat pertussis (whooping cough) is

_____.

15. The incubation period for tetanus is _____ to

_____ days, with the onset commonly occurring at about

_____ days.

WORD LIST

3, 8, 21, fifteenth, eighteenth, airborne, brain damage, cardiac, cyanosis, diphtheria toxoid, droplet, dyspnea, electromyography (EMG), elevated serum creatinine kinase (CK), environmental, erythromycin, folic acid, genetic, good, great vessels, mental retardation, mewing, muscle biopsy, pneumonia, pyloric stenosis, respiratory syncytial virus (RSV), shunt, small, syncope, vitamin A

ANATOMIC STRUCTURES

Label the following anatomic diagrams. For number 2, identify the correct heart defect that each diagram illustrates.

1. Circulation patterns before and after birth

Fetal Circulation

(1) _____

(9) _____

(8) _____

_____

(7) _____

_____

(6) _____

(5) _____

(4) _____

(2) _____

_____

(3) _____

_____

Circulation after Birth

(1) _____

(13) _____

(12) _____

_____

(11) _____

_____

(10) _____

_____

(9) _____

(8) _____

(7) _____

(6) _____

(2) _____

_____

(3) _____

_____

(4) _____

(5) _____

2. Heart defects

PATIENT SCREENING

For each scenario that follows, explain how and why you would schedule an appointment or suggest a referral based on the patient's reported symptoms. First, review the "Guidelines for Patient-Screening Exercises" found on page iii in the "Introduction."

1. The mother of a 6-month-old infant calls the office requesting an appointment for her child. She advises that she thinks the child's head appears swollen and that there are areas that appear to be bulging. What is your response regarding the appointment?

_____

_____

_____

2. The mother of a 3-year-old boy calls to report her child had the onset of vomiting and abdominal pain during the night and is now experiencing blood in his urine. She says she just noticed a swelling on his left side toward his back. She requests an appointment. What is your response regarding the appointment?

_____

_____

_____

3. The mother of a 15-day-old infant son reports that he started having episodes of vomiting with the emesis "shooting out of his mouth" after feeding. She also reports the infant appears hungry, continues to feed, and has not gained any weight. How do you respond to this phone call?

_____

_____

_____

4. Just as the office is closing for the day, a mother calls about her child who just started experiencing signs and symptoms of respiratory distress including hoarseness; fever; a harsh, high-pitched cough; and a funny, high-pitched sound during inspiration. The physician has already left the office for the day. How do you handle this call?

_____

_____

_____

5. A mother calls to report that her three children have been complaining of being fatigued, having headaches, and stomach, muscle, and joint pain for the past 2 weeks. She also states there has been a significant change in their behavior. How do you handle this call?

_____

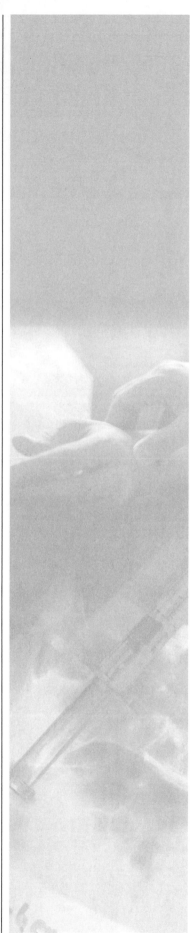

PATIENT TEACHING

*For each scenario that follows, outline the appropriate patient teaching you would perform. **First review** the "Guidelines for Patient-Teaching Exercises" found on page iv in the "Introduction."*

1. SPINA BIFIDA
   Parents have brought the previously diagnosed child to the office for a routine visit. They missed the last regularly scheduled appointment. During the intake assessment, they told you the child had no problems so they did not come. How do you handle this patient (parent)-teaching opportunity?

   _____

   _____

   _____

2. PYLORIC STENOSIS
   An infant has been seen on its first postoperative visit. How do you handle this patient (parent)-teaching opportunity?

   _____

   _____

   _____

3. CHICKENPOX
   A child has just been diagnosed with chickenpox. How do you handle this patient (parent)-teaching opportunity?

   _____

   _____

   _____

4. TONSILLITIS
   A child has just been diagnosed with tonsillitis. The physician has prescribed a round of antibiotics for the child. He has also made note to the parents to ensure that the child has adequate hydration. How do you handle this patient (parent)-teaching opportunity?

   _____

   _____

   _____

5. ASTHMA

A child has been examined for a severe episode of recurring asthma. The physician has prescribed a prophylactic inhalant to be used before exposure. In addition, the child has a prescription for a bronchodilator medication that he is inconsistent in taking. How do you handle this patient (parent)-teaching opportunity?

_____

_____

_____

PHARMACOLOGY QUESTIONS

Circle the letter of the choice that best completes the statement or answers the question.

1. Medications which contain _____ may mask the symptoms of Reye's syndrome and are generally avoided in the treatment of chickenpox.
   a. Acetaminophen
   b. Azithromycin
   c. Aspirin
   d. None of the above.

2. Mumps is a childhood disease which is best prevented by
   a. MMR vaccine.
   b. Gardasil vaccine.
   c. Broad spectrum antibiotics.
   d. None of the above.

3. Acute tonsillitis (strep positive) is generally treated with _____ to prevent rheumatic fever or rheumatic heart disease.
   a. Estradiol (Estrace)
   b. Prednisone
   c. Penicillin
   d. Promethazine

4. Roundworms, pinworms, and tapeworm can be treated with which medication?
   a. Melamine (Antivert)
   b. Finasteride (Proscar)
   c. Mebendazole (Vermox)
   d. Medroxyprogesterone (Provera)

5. Childhood asthma can be treated with all of the following except _____.
   a. Albuterol (Proventil)
   b. Budesonide (Pulmicort)
   c. Tetracycline (Sumycin)
   d. Corticosteroids

Referring to the CDC Childhood and Adolescent Immunization Schedule in the text book answer the following questions:

1. When should an infant receive the first in the series of HepB immunization?

   _____

2. At what age should a child receive the first Varicella immunization?

   _____

3. At what age should a child receive the second MMR?

   _____

4. At what age should a child receive influenza vaccine?

   _____

5. What is the recommended schedule for Hib immunizations?

   _____

ESSAY QUESTION

Write a response to the following question or statement. Use a separate sheet of paper if more space is needed.

Compare the symptoms of the three major types of cerebral palsy: spastic cerebral palsy, athetoid palsy, and ataxic cerebral palsy.

_____

_____

_____

_____

_____

_____

_____

_____

_____

_____

CERTIFICATION EXAMINATION REVIEW

Circle the letter of the choice that best completes the statement or answers the question.

1. Reye's syndrome has been associated with the use of
   a. Acetaminophen.
   b. Ibuprofen.
   c. Aspirin.
   d. All of the above.

2. Loss of appetite, vomiting, irritability, and ataxic gait are symptoms associated with
   a. Muscular dystrophy.
   b. Anemia.
   c. Lead poisoning.
   d. All of the above.

3. The leading cause of absenteeism in school children is
   a. Asthma.
   b. Strep infections.
   c. Bronchitis.
   d. None of the above.

4. The failure of the testicle(s) to descend into the scrotum is called
   a. Cryptorchidism.
   b. Testicular torsion.
   c. Phimosis.
   d. None of the above.

5. If a child is born with tetralogy of Fallot, how many actual heart defects are present?
   a. Two
   b. Three
   c. Four
   d. None of the above

6. When a person is diagnosed with leukemia, there will be a/an
   a. Increase in white blood cells.
   b. Decrease in white blood cells.
   c. Normal white blood cell count.
   d. None of the above.

7. A sensitivity to iron or cow's milk may cause
   a. Cystic fibrosis.
   b. Infantile colic.
   c. Pyloric stenosis.
   d. All of the above.

8. The most progressive form of muscular dystrophy is
   a. Occulta.
   b. Duchenne's.
   c. Down.
   d. None of the above.

9. One way to prevent epidemics of contagious diseases is
   a. Aspirin.
   b. Immunizations.
   c. Multivitamins.
   d. None of the above.

10. Hypertension, hematuria, and pain are symptoms of
    a. Leukemia.
    b. Cystic fibrosis.
    c. Wilms' tumor.
    d. All of the above.

11. The number one cause of death in children between the ages of 1 month to 1 year is
    a. Sudden infant death syndrome.
    b. Cystic fibrosis.
    c. Down syndrome.
    d. Erythroblastosis fetalis.

12. Rheumatic fever, kidney complications, and rheumatic heart disease may be complications of untreated
    a. Lead poisoning.
    b. Tonsillitis caused by A Beta-hemolytic streptococci.
    c. Vomiting and diarrhea.
    d. None of the above.

13. Intracranial pressure is present when cerebrospinal fluid accumulates in the skull when the patient has
    a. Hydrocephalus.
    b. Spina bifida.
    c. Fetal alcohol syndrome.
    d. None of the above.

CHAPTER 3

Immunologic Diseases and Conditions

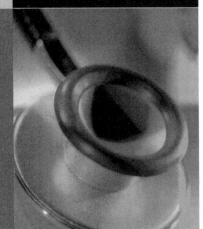

WORD DEFINITIONS

Define the following basic medical terms:

1. Allograft _____

2. Arthralgia _____

3. Conjunctivitis _____

4. Ecchymosis _____

5. Endocrinopathies _____

6. Exacerbate _____

7. Flatulence _____

8. Hypocalcemia _____

9. Lysis _____

10. Neuritis _____

11. Ocular _____

12. Splenomegaly _____

13. Spondylitis _____

14. Stomatitis _____

15. Thyroiditis _____

16. Uveitis _____

17. Vasculitis _____

GLOSSARY TERMS

Define the following chapter glossary terms:

1. Antibodies _____

2. Antigens _____

3. Atrophy _____

4. Autoimmune _____

5. Discoid _____

6. Enzyme-linked immunosorbent assay _____

7. Erythrocyte sedimentation rate (ESR) _____

8. Idiopathic _____

9. Immunocompetent _____

10. Immunodeficiency _____

11. Immunoglobulins _____

12. Immunosuppressive _____

13. Ischemic _____

14. Macrophages _____

15. Megakaryocytes _____

16. Megaloblastic _____

17. Opportunistic infections _____

18. Petechiae _____

19. Phagocytes _____

20. Phagocytosis _____

21. Reticuloendothelial _____

22. Retrovirus _____

23. Tetany _____

24. Thrombocytopenia _____

25. Western blot test _____

SHORT ANSWER

Answer the following questions:

1. What would be included as primary lymphoid tissues?

   _____

2. Which structures are considered the first line of defense against foreign substances or antigens?

   _____

3. Name the two types of acquired specific immunity.

   _____

   _____

4. What is the name of the substance that coats B cells, providing them with the ability to recognize foreign protein, stimulating the antigen-antibody reaction?

   _____

5. What is the name of the virus that causes acquired immunodeficiency syndrome (AIDS)?

   _____

6. Identify the organism responsible for causing a fungal infection of the mucous membranes of the mouth, genitalia, or skin. It is a common opportunistic infection observed in patients who have AIDS.

   _____

7. Is there a cure for AIDS?

   _____

8. Severe combined immunodeficiency (SCID) results from disturbances in the development and function of what cells?

   _____

9. Identify the treatment option for SCID.

   _____

10. When a patient has autoimmune hemolytic anemia, antibodies destroy what?

    _____

11. What is the last treatment used for thrombocytopenic purpura?

    _____

12. What is the name of the fibrous, insoluble protein that is the main component of connective tissue?

   _____

13. Systemic lupus erythematosus is frequently referred to as what?

   _____

14. Name the disease that causes thickening of the skin.

   _____

15. Sjögren's syndrome is more commonly found in families that have what illnesses?

   _____

   _____

16. Name the most severe form of arthritis that commonly causes deformity and disability.

   _____

17. Juvenile rheumatoid arthritis affects children of what ages?

   _____

18. Is ankylosing spondylitis (AS) more prevalent in males or females?

   _____

19. Name the blood tissue antigen that is present in 90% of individuals who have AS.

   _____

20. Cite the body system that is affected when the patient is diagnosed with multiple sclerosis.

   _____

21. Name the drug of choice used to treat myasthenia gravis.

   _____

   _____

22. List examples of organs or tissues that can be successfully transplanted.

   _____

   _____

23. Explain the difference between active and passive immunity.

   _____

24. Discuss the medical management for a patient diagnosed with AIDS.

_____

_____

25. Explain the precautions for immunizing children with Bruton's agammaglobulinemia.

_____

_____

FILL IN THE BLANKS

Fill in the blanks with the correct terms. A word list has been provided. Words used twice are indicated with a (2).

1. The _____ _____ is responsible for a

   complex response to the invasion of the body by foreign substances.

2. Macrophages, which develop from _____, are found in

   the tissues of the liver, lungs, or lymph nodes.

3. If a patient has a positive enzyme-linked immunosorbent assay (ELISA)

   for human immunodeficiency viral (HIV) antibodies, the tests should be

   confirmed with another test called a _____

   _____.

4. Common variable immunodeficiency is an acquired _____

   _____ _____ that results in an absence of

   antibody production or function or both.

5. DiGeorge's anomaly is identified in children who have structural

   anomalies, such as wide-set, downward slanting _____,

   low-set ears with notched _____, a small

   _____, and _____ defects.

6. The mainstay of treatment for chronic mucocutaneous candidiasis is

   _____ agents.

7. The child who has the diagnosis of Wiskott-Aldrich syndrome experiences

   _____ and eczema.

8. Autoimmune diseases occur when _____ develop and

   begin to destroy the body's own _____.

9. Symptoms associated with pernicious anemia include a

_____, _____, _____,

and _____ in the extremities. They may also have

disturbances in digestion as a result of a decrease in the production of

_____ _____.

10. Monthly injections of _____ _____ are

used to treat pernicious anemia.

11. The cause of thrombocytopenic purpura is often considered

_____ although antibodies that reduce the life of

_____ have been found in most cases.

12. Symptoms of Goodpasture syndrome are _____,

_____, relatively acute _____

_____ with _____, anemia hemoptysis,

and _____.

13. Treatment options for collagen diseases are directed at quieting the

overactive _____ _____.

14. The primary objectives of treatment for rheumatoid arthritis are the

_____ of _____ and pain, preservation of

joint _____, and the prevention of joint

_____.

15. The _____ _____ is usually affected by

ankylosing spondylitis.

16. The most common symptom of polymyositis is _____ of

the _____.

17. Prolonged exposure to _____, _____,

_____, and emotional _____ exacerbate

the symptoms of myasthenia gravis.

WORD LIST

acute glomerulonephritis, antifungal, autoantibodies, B cell deficiency, cardiovascular, cells, cold, deformity, eyes, function, hematuria, hydrochloric acid, idiopathic, immune system (2), infections, inflammation, monocytes, mouth, muscles, numbness, pinnas, platelets, proteinuria, reduction, renal failure, sore tongue, spinal column, stress, sunlight, thrombocytopenia, tingling, vitamin B$_{12}$, weakness (2), western blot

ANATOMIC STRUCTURES

Identify the following structures of the immune system.

1. Immune system

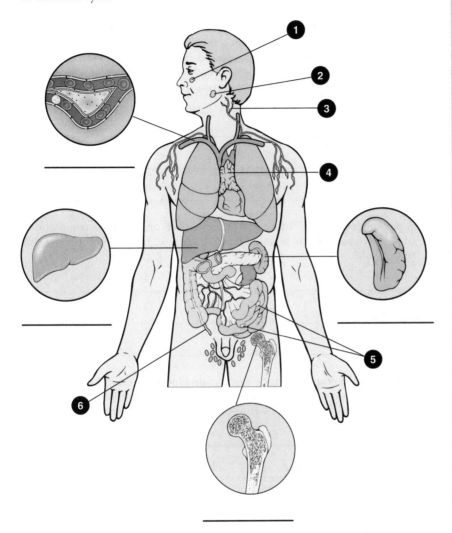

(1) _____   (4) _____

(2) _____   (5) _____

(3) _____   (6) _____

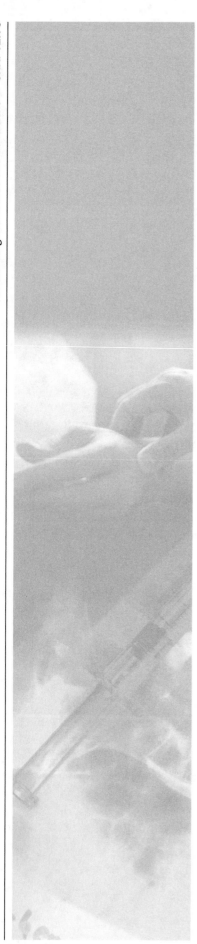

PATIENT SCREENING

For each scenario below, explain how and why you would schedule an appointment or suggest a referral based on the patient's reported symptoms. First, review the "Guidelines for Patient-Screening Exercises" found on page iii in the "Introduction."

1. A woman calls to discuss a condition her husband is experiencing. She reports he is complaining of feeling fatigued and experiencing weakness. Additionally, she tells you he has started experiencing chills, has a fever, and is complaining of shortness of breath. She also states that his skin is pale and jaundiced and that he appears to bruise easily. How do you respond to this phone call?

_____

_____

_____

2. A patient previously diagnosed with pernicious anemia calls complaining of an increased weakness and a rapid heart rate. How do you handle this phone call?

_____

_____

_____

3. A patient calls complaining of spitting up blood, blood in his urine, and a reduced amount of urine. He also mentions a recent weight loss, being fatigued, and having a fever. How do you handle this phone call?

_____

_____

_____

4. The female patient calls stating she is experiencing an unexplained weight loss, fatigue, a persistent low-grade fever, and general malaise. She also mentions joint stiffness, especially on wakening and during periods of inactivity. She is requesting an appointment for an evaluation and treatment of her symptoms. How do you respond to her?

_____

_____

_____

5. A patient has previously been diagnosed with polymyositis. This patient calls the office complaining of a sudden significant loss of strength and some problems swallowing. How do you handle this phone call?

_____

_____

_____

PATIENT TEACHING

For each scenario below, outline the appropriate patient teaching you would perform. First, review the "Guidelines for Patient-Teaching Exercises" found on page iv in the "Introduction."

1. COMMON VARIABLE IMMUNODEFICIENCY (ACQUIRED) HYPOGAMMAGLOBULINEMIA
   Diagnosis of common variable immunodeficiency (acquired) hypo-gammaglobulinemia has just been confirmed. The physician has printed information for patients about this disorder. How do you handle this patient-teaching opportunity?

_____

_____

_____

2. CHRONIC MUCOCUTANEOUS CANDIDIASIS
   A diagnosis of chronic mucocutaneous candidiasis has just been confirmed. The physician has printed material concerning this disorder. You have been instructed to provide this information to the patient and to discuss comfort measures for mouth care. How do you handle this patient-teaching opportunity?

_____

_____

_____

3. IDIOPATHIC THROMBOCYTOPENIC PURPURA
   The child has been diagnosed with idiopathic thrombocytopenic purpura, and infusion therapy is probably going to be prescribed. The physician has printed information regarding this therapy and treatment of this disorder. You are instructed to use this printed information and to discuss it with the family. How do you handle this patient-teaching opportunity?

_____

_____

_____

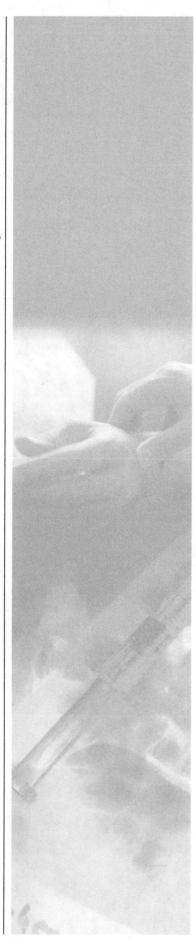

4. **RHEUMATOID ARTHRITIS**

A patient with rheumatoid arthritis has just concluded a visit with the physician. The physician has printed material concerning the cause and treatment options for this disorder. You have been instructed to discuss this material with the patient. How do you handle this patient-teaching opportunity?

_____

_____

_____

5. **MULTIPLE SCLEROSIS**

A patient with multiple sclerosis has experienced an exacerbation of the condition. The physician has printed materials regarding possible treatments of and medications prescribed for this disorder. You are instructed to review this material with the patient. How do you handle this patient-teaching opportunity?

_____

_____

_____

PHARMACOLOGY QUESTIONS

Circle the letter of the choice that best completes the statement or answers the question.

1. Which vitamin is used to treat pernicious anemia?
   a. Vitamin K
   b. Vitamin C
   c. Vitamin E
   d. Vitamin B_{12}

2. Which medications are not used in the treatment of systemic lupus erythematosus?
   a. Antiinflammatory drugs
   b. Anticoagulants
   c. Corticosteroids
   d. Immunosuppressants

3. The drug(s) of choice for myasthenia gravis is (are)
   a. Immunosuppressants.
   b. Corticosteroids.
   c. Mestinon.
   d. None of the above

4. The primary objective of the treatment of rheumatoid arthritis is the reduction of pain and inflammation. Which of the following would be considered first line therapy?
   a. Trazodone (Desyrel)
   b. Antiinflammatory drugs (NSAIDs)
   c. Hormone replacement therapy
   d. Biologic response modifiers

ESSAY QUESTION

Write a response to the following question or statement. Use a separate sheet of paper if more space is needed.

Discuss the guidelines that are included in infection control and Universal Precautions and their importance in the safety of the health care worker.

_____

_____

_____

_____

_____

_____

_____

_____

_____

_____

_____

_____

_____

_____

CERTIFICATION EXAMINATION REVIEW

Circle the letter of the choice that best completes the statement or answers the question.

1. Idiopathic thrombocytopenic anemia involves a deficiency of platelets and
   a. A decrease in red blood cell count.
   b. A decrease in white blood cell count.
   c. The inability of blood to clot.
   d. None of the above.

2. Active immunity is acquired when a person
   a. Has a disease.
   b. Receives an immunization.
   c. Is born.
   d. None of the above

3. Autoimmune diseases occur when
   a. A person's immune system reacts appropriately to an antigen and homeostasis is maintained.
   b. Antibodies develop and begin to destroy the body's own cells.
   c. A person fails to receive childhood immunizations.
   d. All of the above are true.

4. Symptoms of butterfly rash, fever, joint pain, malaise, and weight loss are present with
   a. Scleroderma.
   b. Systemic lupus erythematosus.
   c. Rheumatoid arthritis.
   d. None of the above

5. Symptoms of inflammation and edema are present at the onset of
   a. Scleroderma.
   b. Systemic lupus erythematosus.
   c. Rheumatoid arthritis.
   d. None of the above

6. Symptoms of hardening and shrinking of the skin are associated with
   a. Scleroderma.
   b. Systemic lupus erythematosus.
   c. Rheumatoid arthritis.
   d. None of the above

7. Myasthenia gravis is treated with
   a. Mestinon.
   b. Vitamin B_{12}.
   c. Both a and b.
   d. None of the above

8. The thymus glands produce
   a. A-cell lymphocytes.
   b. C-cell lymphocytes.
   c. T-cell lymphocytes.
   d. All of the above

9. HIV is transmitted by
   a. Close physical contact.
   b. Blood and body fluids.
   c. Both a and b.
   d. None of the above

10. Selective immunoglobulin A deficiency disease is
    a. The most common form of immunodeficiency.
    b. The least common form of immunodeficiency.
    c. Transmitted by close casual contact.
    d. None of the above

11. Pernicious anemia is treated with
    a. Blood transfusions.
    b. Vitamin B_{12}.
    c. Plasma.
    d. None of the above

12. Ankylosing spondylitis primarily affects the
    a. Shoulder.
    b. Spine.
    c. Knee.
    d. All of the above

13. Multiple sclerosis is an inflammatory disease that attacks
    a. The joints.
    b. The spinal nerves.
    c. The myelin sheath.
    d. None of the above

14. Myasthenia gravis is a chronic progressive disease that is characterized by
    a. Muscle stiffness.
    b. Extreme muscular weakness and progressive fatigue.
    c. Pain.
    d. None of the above

15. Congenital X-linked agammaglobulinemia
    a. Is a condition of severe B-cell deficiency.
    b. Affects only males.
    c. Is treated with intravenous infusions of immune globulin.
    d. All of the above

CHAPTER 4

Diseases and Conditions of the Endocrine System

WORD DEFINITIONS

Define the following basic medical terms:

1. Anterior _____

2. Atrophy _____

3. Copious _____

4. Dysfunction _____

5. Encephalopathy _____

6. Fatigue _____

7. Flatus _____

8. Hyperplasia _____

9. Hyposecretion _____

10. Hypotension _____

11. Inspection _____

12. Palpation _____

13. Palpitation _____

14. Polydipsia _____

15. Polyphagia _____

16. Polyuria _____

17. Specific gravity _____

18. Tremor _____

19. Turgor _____

GLOSSARY TERMS

Define the following chapter glossary terms:

1. Adenoma _____

2. Corticotropin _____

3. Dysphagia _____

4. Endemic _____

5. Epiphyseal _____

6. Goitrogenic _____

7. Hyperglycemia _____

8. Hyperlipidemia _____

9. Hyperparathyroidism _____

10. Hypertrophy _____

11. Idiopathic _____

12. Infarct _____

13. Metastasize _____

14. Panhypopituitarism _____

15. Pathogenesis _____

16. Pruritus _____

17. Radioimmunoassay _____

18. Stridor _____

19. Sulfonylureas _____

20. Syncope _____

SHORT ANSWER

Answer the following questions:

1. Name the master gland of the endocrine system.

   _____

2. Identify the hormones responsible for stimulating secretion of other hormones.

   _____

3. Endocrine diseases result from an abnormal secretion of what?

   _____

4. Name three types of laboratory tests that may be used to evaluate hormone levels.

_____

5. Acromegaly and gigantism are conditions resulting from an overproduction of which hormone?

_____

6. Identify the term used for the abnormal underdevelopment of the body occurring in children.

_____

7. Diabetes insipidus is more common in males or females?

_____

8. Name the most common endocrine gland to produce a disease condition or problem.

_____

9. Identify the hormone released from the pituitary gland that controls the activity of the thyroid gland.

_____

10. Is Hashimoto disease more common in male or female patients? Cite statistics of incidence in comparing the sexes.

_____

11. Describe the most outstanding clinical feature of Hashimoto disease.

_____

12. Name the branch of medicine that deals with endocrine disorders.

_____

13. List two examples of ways to ensure ingestion of iodine.

_____

14. Describe the goal of treatment for a patient with Graves' disease.

_____

15. Cite the age range during which cretinism develops.

_____

16. Name the therapeutic agent that is administered to treat myxedema.

_____

17. List the four main types of thyroid cancer.

_____

18. Of the four types, identify the most common type of thyroid cancer.

_____

19. Describe the symptoms of Cushing's syndrome.

_____

_____

20. Explain the treatment for Addison's disease.

_____

_____

_____

21. List five oral medications that are commonly used to treat type 2 diabetes.

_____

22. Name the organs that can be damaged if blood glucose levels are not controlled.

_____

23. Identify the type of diabetes that has its onset during pregnancy.

_____

24. Name the condition associated with a documented low blood glucose level and correlating symptoms that resolve with the administration of glucose.

_____

25. At what age is puberty considered precocious in male adolescents?

_____

26. At what age is puberty considered precocious in female adolescents?

_____

27. Identify the hormone responsible for promoting bone and tissue growth.

_____

28. Identify the hormone responsible for regulating skin pigmentation.

_____

29. Name the hormone that causes uterine contractions.

_____

30. Name the hormone that causes development of female secondary sex characteristics.

_____

FILL IN THE BLANKS

Fill in the blanks with the correct terms. A word list has been provided.

1. The action of most hormones is directed to target _____ or _____ at distant receptor sites, thereby regulating critical body functions such as _____ _____, cellular metabolic rate, and _____ and _____.

2. A frequent cause of an oversecretion of human growth hormone (hGH) is an _____.

3. The cause of hypopituitarism may be a _____ tumor or a tumor of the _____. Some causes are _____ deficiencies. It may also be the result of damage to the _____ gland.

4. The treatment for dwarfism is the administration of _____ until the child reaches the height of 5 feet.

5. Two symptoms of diabetes insipidus are _____ _____ and secretion of _____.

6. A _____ is often the first sign of thyroid disease.

7. The two hormones produced by the thyroid gland are _____ and _____.

8. The cause of Hashimoto disease is unknown, but a _____ _____ is suggested.

9. A patient with Graves' disease exhibits symptoms of _____, nervousness, _____, and _____. There may be other symptoms present in addition to these.

10. A child with cretinism may have symptoms that include _____ and _____ retardation.

11. The face of the patient with _____ becomes bloated, the tongue _____, and the eyelids _____.

12. Thyroid tumors that are undifferentiated, rare, and occur mainly in patients over 60 years of age are _____.

13. Hyperparathyroidism increases the _____ of _____ with the subsequent release of _____ _____ and extracellular fluid.

14. The patient with Addison's disease would exhibit elevated serum _____, blood urea nitrogen, _____ and eosinophil levels, and elevated _____.

15. Patients with type _____ diabetes do not usually require insulin to control blood glucose levels.

16. Thirty to _____ percent of women who have had gestational diabetes mellitus (GDM) develop type 2 diabetes within 5 to 10 years after giving birth.

17. An individual with severe symptoms of _____ _____ hypoglycemia requires _____ medical attention.

18. Precocious puberty in the male adolescent is exhibited by early development of _____ _____ characteristics, _____ development, and spermatogenesis.

19. In most cases the cause of precocious puberty in females is _____ without associated abnormalities.

20. The hormone responsible for initiating growth of eggs in the ovaries and stimulating spermatogenesis in the testes is called _____ _____ _____.

WORD LIST

acute reactive, anaplastic, anterior pituitary adenoma, bone, 2, breakdown, congenital, damage, dilute urine, emergency, excessive calcium, excitability, extreme thirst, follicle stimulating hormone, forty, genetic factor, glands, goiter, gonadal, growth, growth and development, hematocrit, hypothalamus, idiopathic, insomnia, lymphocyte, mental, myxedema, palpitations, pituitary, potassium, puffy, rapid heartbeat, secondary sex, somatotropin (hGH), thick, thyroxine (T_4), tissues, tri-iodothyronine (T_3), urinary output

ANATOMIC STRUCTURES

Identify the following structures of the endocrine system.

1. Major glands of the normal endocrine system

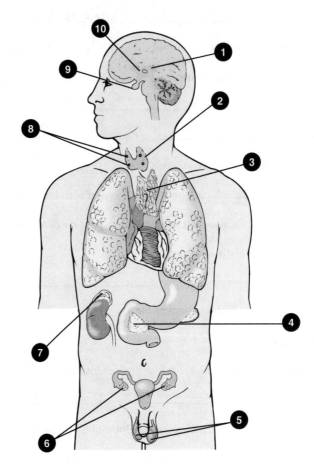

(1) _____

(2) _____

(3) _____

(4) _____

(5) _____

(6) _____

(7) _____

(8) _____

(9) _____

(10) _____

PATIENT SCREENING

For each scenario below, explain how and why you would schedule an appointment or suggest a referral based on the patient's reported symptoms. First, review the "Guidelines for Patient-Screening Exercises" found on page iii in the "Introduction."

1. A male patient calls for an appointment. He reports experiencing the sudden onset of excessive thirst and urination. He says that he is thirsty all the time and cannot seem to get enough to drink. How do you respond to this phone call?

_____

_____

_____

2. A female patient calls the office and says she thinks she has swelling in her neck and is beginning to experience difficulty swallowing. How do you respond to this phone call?

_____

_____

_____

3. An individual calls the office stating he is experiencing periods of rapid heartbeat and palpitations, insomnia, nervousness, and excitability. He states that despite excessive appetite and food ingestion, he is losing weight. How do you respond to this call?

_____

_____

_____

4. A woman calls the office stating that her husband, who has been diagnosed with diabetes, is experiencing excessive thirst, nausea, drowsiness, and abdominal pain. She just noticed a fruity odor on his breath. She wants to know what to do. How do you respond to this call?

_____

_____

_____

5. A patient calls the office saying she has started experiencing weight loss, excessive thirst, excessive hunger, and frequent urination. She also tells you her mother and aunt have diabetes. She says she just does not feel right. How do you respond to this call?

_____

_____

_____

PATIENT TEACHING

For each scenario that follows, outline the appropriate patient teaching you would perform. First, review the "Guidelines for Patient-Teaching Exercises" found on page iv in the "Introduction."

1. ACROMEGALY
   A diagnosis of acromegaly has been confirmed. The physician (an endocrinologist) has printed materials concerning the disorder. You have been instructed to review the material with the patient and his or her family. How do you handle this patient-teaching opportunity?

   _____

   _____

   _____

2. DIABETES INSIPIDUS
   A diagnosis of diabetes insipidus has been confirmed. You are instructed to use available printed material to discuss treatment guidelines with the patient. How do you handle this patient-teaching opportunity?

   _____

   _____

   _____

3. GRAVES' DISEASE
   An individual with Graves' disease has been noncompliant with prescribed medications and has experienced an exacerbation of the condition. The physician has decided the patient requires additional information about the disorder. You are instructed to review the printed materials and guidelines with the patient. How do you handle this patient-teaching opportunity?

   _____

   _____

   _____

4. HYPOTHYROIDISM

A diagnosis of hypothyroidism has just been confirmed. The physician has prescribed a thyroid replacement drug with instructions to take the medication as directed and to schedule a checkup in 6 weeks. Additionally, the patient has been told to contact the physician if he or she experiences a rapid heartbeat. How do you handle this patient-teaching opportunity?

_____

_____

_____

5. DIABETES MELLITUS

A previously diagnosed individual with diabetes mellitus has been having difficulty maintaining therapeutic glucose levels. You are instructed to provide instructional material concerning the importance of monitoring glucose levels and possible complications of the disorder. How would you handle this patient-teaching opportunity?

_____

_____

_____

PHARMACOLOGY QUESTIONS

Circle the letter of the choice that best completes the statement or answers the question.

1. Hypothyroidism is usually treated with thyroid replacement hormones. Which of the following is not a type of thyroid replacement?
   a. Levothyroxine (Synthroid)
   b. Armour thyroid
   c. Extropiate (Estrace)
   d. None of the above

2. Type 2 diabetes can be treated with all of the following therapies except
   a. Diet and exercise.
   b. Corticosteroids.
   c. Sulfonylurea drugs.
   d. Insulin.

3. Type 1 diabetes can be treated with all of the following therapies except
   a. Short-acting insulin.
   b. Long-acting insulin.
   c. Inhaled insulin.
   d. None of the above

4. If a patient tests his blood glucose level and it is very high (over 300), what would be the fastest way to reduce his blood glucose level?
   a. Insulin
   b. A simple sugar
   c. Metformin (Glucophage)
   d. Proglitizone (Precose)

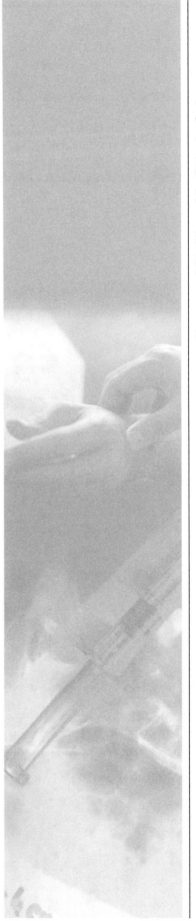

ESSAY QUESTION

Write a response to the following question or statement. Use a separate sheet of paper if more space is needed.

Explain the symptoms and treatment for hypoglycemia. Why is this condition considered serious?

_____

_____

_____

_____

_____

_____

_____

_____

_____

_____

_____

_____

_____

_____

CERTIFICATION EXAMINATION REVIEW

Circle the letter of the choice that best completes the statement or answers the question.

1. Acromegaly is caused from a hypersecretion of human growth hormone (hGH) that occurs
   a. After puberty.
   b. Before puberty.
   c. At birth.
   d. None of the above

2. Inadequate amounts of dietary iodine may be the cause of
   a. Graves' disease.
   b. A simple nontoxic goiter.
   c. Addison's disease.
   d. None of the above

3. A calculated diet and exercise, blood and urine testing, and insulin administration are treatments for
   a. Gestational diabetes.
   b. Diabetes insipidus.
   c. Diabetes mellitus.
   d. None of the above

4. Hyperglycemia, thirst, nausea, vomiting, and dry skin are all symptoms of
   a. Diabetic coma.
   b. Insulin shock.
   c. Gestational diabetes.
   d. None of the above

5. Any dysfunction of the endocrine system may result in a/an
   a. Increase secretion of hormones.
   b. Decrease in secretion of hormones.
   c. Both of the above
   d. None of the above

6. A conscious person experiencing insulin shock requires
   a. Insulin.
   b. Glucose.
   c. Simple sugar.
   d. None of the above

7. Severe hypothyroidism or myxedema has its onset during
   a. Infancy.
   b. Older childhood.
   c. Adulthood.
   d. Both b and c

8. Dwarfism is the abnormal underdevelopment of the body or hypopituitarism that occurs in
   a. Infancy.
   b. Older childhood.
   c. Adulthood.
   d. None of the above

9. Gigantism is caused from a hypersecretion of human growth hormone that occurs
   a. Before puberty.
   b. After puberty.
   c. At any age.
   d. At birth.

10. Cushing's syndrome causes symptoms of
    a. Weight loss, rash, and alopecia.
    b. Fatigue, muscle weakness, and changes in body appearance.
    c. A bright red rash and itching.
    d. None of the above

11. Palpation of a hard, painless lump or nodule on the thyroid gland, vocal cord paralysis, obstructive symptoms, and cervical-lymph adenopathy all indicate
    a. An evaluation for cancer of the thyroid gland.
    b. A diagnosis of Cushing's syndrome.
    c. A diagnosis of acromegaly.
    d. None of the above

12. Addison's disease has a gradual onset and involves the
    a. Parathyroid glands.
    b. Pancreas.
    c. Adrenal glands.
    d. Thyroid gland.

CHAPTER 5

Diseases and Disorders of the Eye and Ear

WORD DEFINITIONS

Define the following basic medical terms:

1. Arteritis _____

2. Bilateral _____

3. Dilated _____

4. Edema _____

5. Excision _____

6. Hemorrhage _____

7. Hyperopia _____

8. Hypertrophied _____

9. Intracranial _____

10. Intraocular _____

11. Meningitis _____

12. Myopia _____

13. Postoperative _____

14. Proliferative _____

15. Strabismus _____

16. Systemic _____

17. Topical _____

18. Vertigo _____

GLOSSARY TERMS

Define the following chapter glossary terms:

1. Amblyopia _____

2. Analgesics _____

3. Ankylosis _____

4. Audiogram _____

5. Diplopia _____

6. Histoplasmosis _____

7. Laser
   photocoagulation _____

8. Macula _____

9. Photophobia _____

10. Purulent _____

11. Seborrhea _____

12. Tinnitus _____

13. Tonometry _____

14. Toxoplasmosis _____

15. Tympanic
    membrane _____

SHORT ANSWER

Answer the following questions:

1. Identify the concentric layers of the eyeball that are its primary structure.

   _____

2. Name the colorless transparent structure located on the front of the eye.

   _____

3. List the way that hearing loss is classified.

   _____

4. Explain the symptoms associated with otosclerosis.

   _____

5. Name the canal that leads from the middle ear to the nasopharynx.

_____

6. Identify the structure in the ear that is responsible for helping a person maintain balance.

_____

7. Cite the shape of the normal eyeball.

_____

8. Name the sensory receptive cells in the retina that make the detection of color and fine detail possible.

_____

9. Identify the waxlike secretion that is produced by the glands of the external ear canal.

_____

10. Name the jellylike fluid found in the cavity behind the lens of the eye.

_____

11. Name the internal elastic structure of the eye that focuses images both near and far.

_____

12. What is the cause of a cholesteatoma?

_____

13. If the eyeball is abnormally short, name the condition that occurs.

_____

14. If the eyeball is abnormally long, name the condition that occurs.

_____

15. Identify the cause of astigmatism.

_____

16. List the primary symptoms of refractive errors.

_____

17. Name the most common type of nystagmus.

_____

18. Identify the bacteria that are the common cause of styes.

_____

19. List the symptoms of keratitis.

_____

20. Explain the most common cause of cataracts.

_____

21. Is there a cure for macular degeneration?

_____

22. Identify the disorder of the retinal blood vessels that may develop in a person who has diabetes.

_____

23. Explain the steps that may be used to remove impacted cerumen.

_____

_____

24. List the four most common causes of a ruptured eardrum.

_____

_____

FILL IN THE BLANKS

Fill in the blanks with the correct terms. A word list has been provided. Words used twice are indicated with a (2).

1. The iris or colored portion of the eye helps regulate the amount of

   _____ that enters the eye.

2. The large cavity behind the lens of the eye contains a jellylike fluid called

   the _____.

3. Four main refractive errors that result when the eye is unable to

   focus light effectively on the retina are _____,

   _____, _____, and _____.

4. The patient with myopia can see objects that are near, but experiences

   difficulty seeing objects that are _____.

5. _____ is the failure of the eyes to look in the same

   direction at the same time, which primarily occurs because of

   _____ in the nerves stimulating the muscles that control

   the _____ of the eye.

6. In _____, both eyes turn inward; in exotropia, both eyes turn outward.

7. The symptoms of a stye are _____, _____, _____, and formation of pus at the site.

8. Keratitis is frequently caused by an infection resulting from the _____ _____ virus.

9. Allergies or exposure to _____, dust, or _____ can cause nonulcerative blepharitis.

10. Blepharoptosis occurs at any _____, is often _____, and if severe, blocks the _____ of the affected eye.

11. Infection, either _____ or _____, can cause conjunctivitis.

12. A corneal abrasion is the painful loss of _____ epithelium, or outer layer of the _____.

13. A cataract may become visible, giving the pupil a _____, opaque appearance.

14. The best way to detect glaucoma is to have periodic _____ _____ examinations.

15. Common symptoms of ear diseases and conditions that should receive medical attention include _____ _____, ear _____ or _____, _____, vertigo, nausea, and _____.

16. Impacted _____ may harden and block sound waves resulting in decreased hearing.

17. Otitis _____ is the most frequent reason for visits to the physician by children.

WORD LIST

age, astigmatism, bacterial, cerumen, chemicals, cornea, distant, esotropia, familial, hearing loss, herpes simplex, hyperopia, light, media, myopia, pain (2), position, presbyopia, pressure, routine ophthalmic, redness, smoke, strabismus, surface, swelling, tinnitus, viral, vision, vitreous humor, vomiting, weakness, white

ANATOMIC STRUCTURES

Identify the structures in the following anatomic diagrams.

1. Normal eye

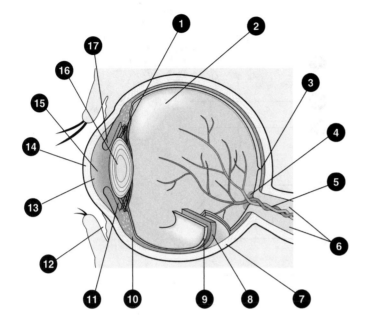

(1) _____

(2) _____

(3) _____

(4) _____

(5) _____

(6) _____

(7) _____

(8) _____

(9) _____

(10) _____

(11) _____

(12) _____

(13) _____

(14) _____

(15) _____

(16) _____

(17) _____

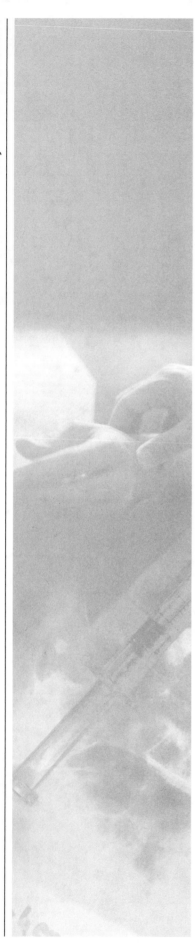

2. The visual pathway

Left visual field   Right visual field

Temporal   Temporal

Nasal

Left eye   Right eye

1
2
3
4
5

(1) _____

(2) _____

(3) _____

(4) _____

(5) _____

3. Normal ear

(1) _____

(2) _____

(3) _____

(4) _____

(5) _____

(6) _____

(7) _____

(8) _____

(9) _____

(10) _____

(11) _____

(12) _____

4. Labyrinth or inner ear

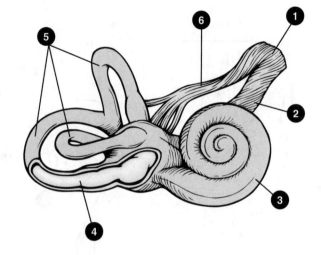

(1) _____

(2) _____

(3) _____

(4) _____

(5) _____

(6) _____

PATIENT SCREENING

For each scenario that follows, explain how and why you would schedule an appointment or suggest a referral based on the patient's reported symptoms. First, review the "Guidelines for Patient-Screening Exercises" found on page iii in the "Introduction."

1. A patient calls in describing a sensation of constantly having something in her right eye. She also states the pain and tearing prevent her from wearing her contact lens in that eye. How do you handle this call?

_____

_____

_____

2. A patient calls in advising he is experiencing changes in his vision and a sensitivity to light. How do you handle this call?

_____

_____

_____

3. A patient calls in reporting she is experiencing reduced vision, especially loss of sharpness in her central vision. How do you respond to this call?

_____

_____

_____

_____

4. A patient calls the office and tells you he suddenly is having flashes of light along with floating spots in the left eye. How do you respond to this call?

_____

_____

_____

_____

5. A father calls the office reporting his child is experiencing ear pain, has a fever, and appears to have diminished hearing. How do you handle this call?

_____

_____

_____

_____

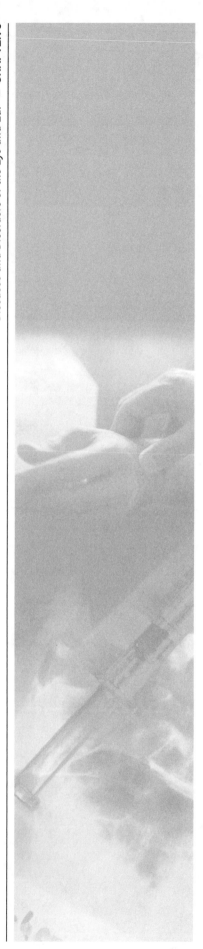

PATIENT TEACHING

For each scenario below, outline the appropriate patient teaching you would perform. First, review the "Guidelines for Patient-Teaching Exercises" found on page iv in the "Introduction."

1. STYE

   A patient has just been diagnosed with having a stye on the eyelid. Eye compresses and topical antibiotics have been prescribed. You are instructed to provide the patient with instructions regarding the application of compresses and topical eye medications. How would you handle this patient-teaching opportunity?

   _____

   _____

   _____

   _____

2. KERATITIS

   A diagnosis of keratitis has been made. The physician instructs you to use printed materials to explain proper administration of eye medications and to reinforce the importance of good hand washing before touching an eye. How do you handle this patient-teaching opportunity?

   _____

   _____

   _____

   _____

3. CONJUNCTIVITIS

   A patient with conjunctivitis has been advised to use cool compresses on both eyes for comfort. Topical ophthalmic medications have also been prescribed for therapeutic treatment. You have been instructed to advise the patient on how to apply the cool compresses and medications. How would you handle this patient-teaching opportunity?

   _____

   _____

   _____

   _____

4. GLAUCOMA

   A patient has just been diagnosed with glaucoma. (Type is insignificant in this situation.) You have been instructed to discuss treatment regimen with the patient. How do you handle this patient-teaching opportunity?

   _____

   _____

   _____

   _____

5. IMPACTED CERUMEN

   A child has been experiencing diminished hearing and has been complaining of slight pain in the ears. A diagnosis of impacted cerumen is made. You are instructed to reinforce appropriate cleansing of the ear canal. How do you handle this patient-teaching opportunity?

   _____

   _____

   _____

   _____

PHARMACOLOGY QUESTIONS

Circle the letter of the choice that best completes the statement or answers the question.

1. Treatment of more severe blepharitis may include which of the following?
   a. Oral indomethacin
   b. Antibiotic ophthalmic ointment
   c. Conjugated estrogen (Premarin)
   d. Terbinafine ointment (Bactroban)

2. Bacterial conjunctivitis is best treated with _____.
   a. Clopidogrel
   b. Clotrimazole (Lotrimin)
   c. Topical antibiotics
   d. Prednisone

3. Which of the following medications can be used for the treatment of glaucoma?
   a. Betaxolol (Betagan)
   b. Timolol (Timoptic)
   c. Latanoprost (Xalatan)
   d. All of the above.

4. In order to achieve best results in the treatment of open angle glaucoma, the patient should be instructed to _____.
   a. Apply cold compresses to the eye twice a day.
   b. Use the prescribed eye medication on a regular basis and not miss doses
   c. Use the prescribed eye medication only if headache or blurred vision is present
   d. None of the above.

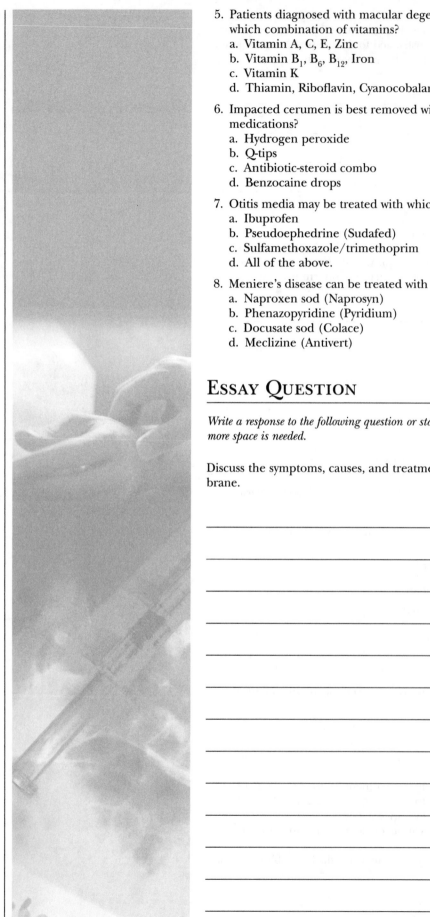

5. Patients diagnosed with macular degeneration are commonly prescribed which combination of vitamins?
   a. Vitamin A, C, E, Zinc
   b. Vitamin B_1, B_6, B_{12}, Iron
   c. Vitamin K
   d. Thiamin, Riboflavin, Cyanocobalamin

6. Impacted cerumen is best removed with which of the following medications?
   a. Hydrogen peroxide
   b. Q-tips
   c. Antibiotic-steroid combo
   d. Benzocaine drops

7. Otitis media may be treated with which medication?
   a. Ibuprofen
   b. Pseudoephedrine (Sudafed)
   c. Sulfamethoxazole/trimethoprim
   d. All of the above.

8. Meniere's disease can be treated with which of the following medications?
   a. Naproxen sod (Naprosyn)
   b. Phenazopyridine (Pyridium)
   c. Docusate sod (Colace)
   d. Meclizine (Antivert)

Essay Question

Write a response to the following question or statement. Use a separate sheet of paper if more space is needed.

Discuss the symptoms, causes, and treatment for a ruptured tympanic membrane.

_____

_____

_____

_____

_____

_____

_____

_____

_____

_____

_____

_____

CERTIFICATION EXAMINATION REVIEW

Circle the letter of the choice that best completes the statement or answers the question.

1. When the eye is unable to focus light effectively, which of the following may result?
   a. Hyperopia
   b. Myopia
   c. Presbyopia
   d. All of the above

2. Laser surgery, contact lenses, and eyeglasses would be treatment for
   a. Folliculitis.
   b. Conjunctivitis.
   c. Refractive errors.
   d. All of the above.

3. A stye is an
   a. Inflammation of the conjunctiva.
   b. Inflammation of the sebaceous glands of the eyelid.
   c. Inflammation of the retina.
   d. None of the above

4. Conjunctivitis is an
   a. Inflammation of the conjunctiva, the mucous membrane that covers the anterior portion of the eyeball and also lines the eyelid.
   b. Inflammation of the hair follicle of the eyelid.
   c. Inflammation of the retina.
   d. None of the above

5. Infection, irritation, allergies, or chemicals may be the cause of
   a. Hyperopia.
   b. Myopia.
   c. Conjunctivitis.
   d. All of the above

6. Glaucoma is a major cause of _____ in the United States.
   a. Blindness
   b. Hearing loss
   c. Retinal detachment
   d. None of the above

7. Otosclerosis is an ankylosing of the
   a. Labyrinth.
   b. Stapes.
   c. Eyelid.
   d. None of the above

8. Labyrinthitis is an inflammation of the
   a. Stapes.
   b. Conjunctiva.
   c. Semicircular canal.
   d. None of the above

9. Otosclerosis, impacted cerumen, and otitis media may be the etiology of
   a. Conductive hearing loss.
   b. Sensorineural hearing loss.
   c. Both a and b.
   d. Neither a nor b.

10. The internal _____ of the eye is elastic and can focus images both near and far.
    a. Sclera
    b. Iris
    c. Lens
    d. None of the above

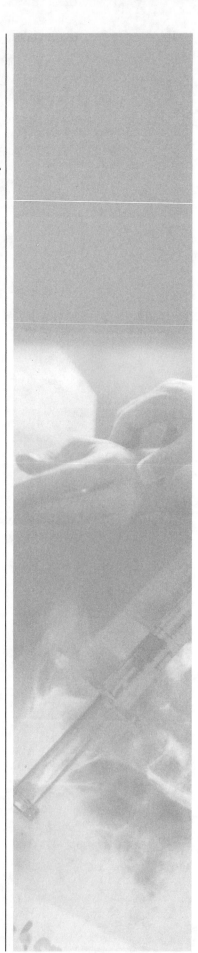

11. The *most common* cause of blindness in the United States is
    a. Uveitis.
    b. Retinal detachment.
    c. Macular degeneration.
    d. Cataract.

CHAPTER 6

Diseases and Conditions of the Integumentary System

WORD DEFINITIONS

Define the following basic medical terms:

1. Albinism _____

2. Colic _____

3. Edema _____

4. Epidemic _____

5. Erythema _____

6. Excision _____

7. Hyperplastic _____

8. Hypertrophic _____

9. Lesion _____

10. Peripheral _____

11. Psychosis _____

12. Sebaceous _____

13. Spore _____

14. Superficial _____

15. Unilateral _____

GLOSSARY TERMS

Define the following chapter glossary terms:

1. Asymptomatic
2. Comedones
3. Debriding
4. Dermatomes
5. Exacerbations
6. Idiopathic
7. Keratin
8. Keratolytic
9. Melanin
10. Papules
11. Plaques
12. Pustules
13. Sebum
14. Toxic
15. Vesicles

SHORT ANSWER

Answer the following questions:

1. List the functions of the skin.

2. Describe the symptoms of psoriasis.

3. Identify the oily secretion that is produced by the sebaceous glands.

4. How are diagnoses of cutaneous diseases based?

5. Identify another name for a skin tag.

6. Which type of skin cancer is the most prevalent form of cancer worldwide?

_____

7. Identify the bacteria that cause impetigo.

_____

8. List examples of dermatophytosis.

_____

9. List examples of common benign skin tumors.

_____

10. Identify the other name for a mole.

_____

11. Are keloids benign or malignant?

_____

12. When do keloids form?

_____

13. At what age will cradle cap resolve if left untreated?

_____

14. Name the test that is used to identify specific irritants or allergens that cause contact dermatitis.

_____

15. List three things that may cause eczema to flare up.

_____

16. Explain the goal of treatment for psoriasis.

_____

17. Identify the other name for herpes zoster.

_____

18. Cite the other name for a furuncle.

_____

19. Which area of the body is usually affected by cellulitis?

_____

20. Describe the appearance of a ringworm lesion.

_____

21. Identify the area of the body affected by tinea unguium.

_____

22. Identify the area of the body affected by tinea pedis.

_____

23. Which sex is more at risk for tinea cruris?

_____

24. Cite the statistics for lesion occurrence of basal cell carcinoma on the face.

_____

25. Cite the statistics for 5-year survival rate of nonmelanoma skin cancer.

_____

26. Name the special cells in the skin that produce melanin.

_____

27. What color eyes would a person with albinism have?

_____

28. Will alopecia resulting from the aging process or heredity improve?

_____

29. State the cause of warts.

_____

30. List some of the likely causes of deformed or discolored nails.

_____

FILL IN THE BLANKS

Fill in the blanks with the correct terms. A word list has been provided.

1. The skin is one of the _____ organs in size.

2. The dermis is the _____ layer of the skin.

3. The _____ is the outer thin layer of the skin that

   is responsible for the production of _____ and

   _____.

4. The third layer of the skin is the _____, a thick, fat-containing section that provides _____ for the body against heat loss.

5. Seborrheic dermatitis can be treated effectively with topical _____ cream.

6. Urticaria, or _____, is associated with symptoms of severe _____, followed by the appearance of _____ and an area of swelling.

7. Albinism is a rare _____ condition.

8. Melasma occurs in some women during _____ changes. The condition disappears after _____ or when oral contraceptive use is _____.

9. Hemangiomas are _____ lesions of proliferating _____ that produce a _____, blue, or _____ color.

10. Seborrheic _____ are not true warts but are _____ or oval patches of _____ pigmented skin.

11. A fungal infection that causes patches of flaky light or dark skin to develop on the trunk of the body is called _____.

12. The treatment that is showing promise for male pattern baldness is _____ preparations used topically in cream and spray forms.

WORD LIST

benign, blood vessels, discontinued, epidermis, hives, hormonal, hydro-cortisone, inherited, insulation, itching, keratin, largest, melanin, middle, minoxidil (Rogaine), pityriasis, pregnancy, purple, red, redness, round, subcutaneous layer, warts

ANATOMIC STRUCTURES

Identify the structures of the following anatomic diagram.

1. Normal skin

(1) _____ (11) _____

(2) _____ (12) _____

(3) _____ (13) _____

(4) _____ (14) _____

(5) _____ (15) _____

(6) _____ (16) _____

(7) _____ (17) _____

(8) _____ (18) _____

(9) _____ (19) _____

(10) _____

PATIENT SCREENING

For each scenario below, explain how and why you would schedule an appointment or suggest a referral based on the patient's reported symptoms. First, review the "Guidelines for Patient-Screening Exercises" found on page iii in the "Introduction."

1. The mother of a 10-year-old child calls in to request an appointment for her daughter who has seeping eruptions on her elbows and knees. She also says the child is experiencing constant itching. How do you handle this phone call?

_____

_____

_____

2. A patient calls complaining of severe itching of the arms, hands, and trunk that is accompanied by a red rash. This situation has occurred in the past 2 hours and is getting progressively worse. How do you handle this call?

_____

_____

_____

3. A patient's wife calls in stating her husband has the onset of excruciating pain on the right side in the middle of the trunk. She says it appears there are small blisterlike eruptions over the area on the right side of the body. She says he needs help as soon as possible. How do you handle this call?

_____

_____

_____

4. A mother calls reporting her daughter has just come home from school with areas on her legs and arms having small blisters that are surrounded with small blisterlike formations. She says the child is continuously scratching the areas, and they are getting worse. She requests an appointment for the next morning, saying she will keep the child home from school until seen by the physician. When do you schedule the child to be seen?

_____

_____

_____

5. A female patient calls stating she has a sore on her right shoulder that has refused to heal completely and has occurrences of bleeding. She states that the sore is about an inch in diameter and has irregular edges. She requests an appointment for assessment of the sore. How do you schedule the appointment?

_____

_____

_____

PATIENT TEACHING

For each scenario below, outline the appropriate patient teaching you would perform. First, review the "Guidelines for Patient-Teaching Exercises" found on page iv in the "Introduction."

1. CONTACT DERMATITIS
   A patient has just been seen for the second time in 3 weeks for contact dermatitis. The area is now showing signs of a developing infection. The physician instructs you to reinforce his instructions about avoiding the trigger substance and trying to avoid scratching the area. How do you handle the patient-teaching opportunity?

   _____

   _____

   _____

2. ACNE
   A teenage patient has experienced an exacerbation of acne. Topical and oral medications have been prescribed. You have been instructed to provide the patient with printed information regarding the treatment of acne. How do you handle this patient-teaching opportunity?

   _____

   _____

   _____

3. DERMATOPHYTOSIS
   A patient has been diagnosed with athlete's foot. You have been instructed to provide him or her with printed information regarding the treatment of this condition. How do you handle this patient-teaching opportunity?

   _____

   _____

   _____

4. SCABIES AND PEDICULOSIS

A patient was sent home from school with the possibility of head lice. You have been instructed to provide the parents and patient with printed information regarding this condition. How will you handle this patient-teaching opportunity?

_____

_____

_____

5. SKIN CANCER

A patient has been seen for several skin lesions. Some are diagnosed as being benign. One is suspicious in nature, and the patient is referred to a dermatologist for further assessment and treatment. You are instructed to provide the patient with printed information concerning skin lesions and to encourage the use of sunscreen. How do you handle this patient-teaching opportunity?

_____

_____

_____

PHARMACOLOGY QUESTIONS

Circle the letter of the choice that best completes the statement or answers the question.

1. Which of the following medications is not used to treat atopic dermatitis (eczema)?
   a. Diazepam (Valium)
   b. Diphenhydramine (Benadryl)
   c. Tacrolimus (Protopic)
   d. Disopyramide (Norpace)

2. Acne vulgaris may be treated with _____?
   a. Tretinoin (Retin-A)
   b. Antibiotics
   c. Isotretinoin (Accutane)
   d. All of the above.

3. Antiviral therapy is commonly used to treat shingles. Which of the following is not an antiviral medication?
   a. Acyclovir (Zovirax)
   b. Capsaicin (Zostrix)
   c. Famciclovir (Famvir)
   d. Valacyclovir (Valtrex)

4. If treating a patient with a case of impetigo, which antibiotic would be best?
   a. Penicillin
   b. Metronidazole (Flagyl)
   c. Mupirocin (Bactroban)
   d. Tetracycline

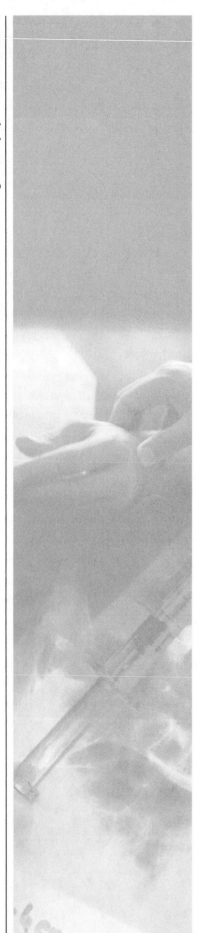

5. Which of the following would not be used for the treatment of cellulitis ?
   a. Penicillin
   b. Acetaminophen (Tylenol)
   c. Codeine
   d. Medroxyprogesterone (Provera)

6. Ringworm (tinea corporis) is treated with which of the following?
   a. Permethrin (Elimite)
   b. Mebendazole (Vermox)
   c. Pyrantel (Pin X)
   d. Terbinafine (Lamisil)

7. Head lice can be treated with which of the following?
   a. Lindane shampoo
   b. Fine tooth comb
   c. Permethrin (Elimite)
   d. All of the above.

ESSAY QUESTION

Write a response to the following question or statement. Use a separate sheet of paper if more space is needed.

Describe the cause, symptoms, and treatment for herpes zoster (shingles).

_____

_____

_____

_____

_____

_____

_____

_____

_____

_____

CERTIFICATION EXAMINATION REVIEW

Circle the letter of the choice that best completes the statement or answers the question.

1. Streptococcus or Staphylococcus are bacteria that can cause the skin infection called
   a. Psoriasis.
   b. Eczema.
   c. Impetigo.
   d. None of the above.

2. Atopic dermatitis is another name for _____. This is a skin infection that tends to occur in people who have a family history of allergic conditions.
   a. Psoriasis
   b. Eczema
   c. Impetigo
   d. None of the above.

3. Cradle cap is a type of seborrheic dermatitis that is seen in
   a. Infants.
   b. Teenagers.
   c. Adults.
   d. All of the above.

4. Good skin care, early ambulation, position changes every 2 hours are all considered preventative measures to reduce the likelihood of developing _____ _____.
   a. Herpes zoster
   b. Decubitus ulcers
   c. Atopic dermatitis
   d. None of the above

5. The two most common parasitic infections to infest man are
   a. Herpes zoster.
   b. Atopic dermatitis.
   c. Scabies and pediculosis.
   d. None of the above.

6. Malignant melanoma is the most serious type of
   a. Skin cancer.
   b. Fungal infection.
   c. Parasitic infection.
   d. None of the above.

7. A furuncle is an abscess that involves the entire hair follicle and
   a. Underlying muscle tissue.
   b. The epidermis.
   c. The adjacent subcutaneous tissue.
   d. None of the above.

8. Manifestations of dermatophytosis include
   a. Tinea capitis, tinea corporis, tinea pedis and tinea cruris.
   b. Scabies and pediculosis.
   c. Albinism and vitiligo.
   d. All of the above.

9. The patient with psoriasis will exhibit symptoms of
   a. A fine red rash that itches.
   b. Large furuncles and a fine red rash.
   c. Thick, flaky red patches of various sizes, covered with white silvery scales.
   d. None of the above.

10. The transmission of lice and scabies from one person to another is
    a. Difficult.
    b. Easy with close physical contact.
    c. Only possible if two people live in the same house.
    d. None of the above.

CHAPTER 7

Diseases and Conditions of the Musculoskeletal System

WORD DEFINITIONS

Define the following basic medical terms:

1. Adjacent _____

2. Bacterium _____

3. Bunionectomy _____

4. Calcanean _____

5. Calcification _____

6. Collagen _____

7. Edematous _____

8. Extension _____

9. Fasciitis _____

10. Flexion _____

11. Hyperbaric
    oxygen treatment _____

12. Hyperostosis _____

13. Intraarticular _____

14. Laxity _____

15. Osteotomy _____

16. Plantar _____

GLOSSARY TERMS

Define the following chapter glossary terms:

1. Abscess _____

2. Arthrodesis _____

3. Arthroplasty _____

4. Cheilectomy _____

5. Closed reduction _____

6. Echocardiographic _____

7. Hallux _____

8. Hyperuricemia _____

9. Magnetic resonance imaging (MRI) _____

10. Metatarsophalangeal _____

11. Open reduction _____

12. Osteophytes _____

13. Periosteum _____

14. Purulent _____

15. Sclerosing _____

16. Sequestrum _____

17. Skeletal traction _____

18. Subluxation _____

19. Synovial _____

20. Tendinitis _____

SHORT ANSWER

Answer the following questions:

1. Identify when shin splints are likely to occur.

_____

2. Cite the cause of fibromyalgia.

_____

3. Is there a specific laboratory test to identify whether a patient has fibromyalgia?

_____

4. Name the most common form of arthritis.

_____

5. Describe the rash that sometimes accompanies Lyme disease.

_____

6. Identify the cause of gouty arthritis.

_____

7. Name the hereditary syndrome that affects the connective tissue and causes an abnormal growth of the extremities.

_____

8. Cite the other name for Paget's disease.

_____

9. Identify the most common sites of the body affected by Paget's disease.

_____

10. Name the most common type of primary bone neoplasm.

_____

11. A deficiency in vitamin D may cause what abnormal metabolic bone disease?

_____

12. Which sex is more likely to be affected by osteoporosis?

_____

13. Name the term for a benign growth filled with a jellylike substance that commonly develops on the back of the wrist and may be caused by repetitive injury.

_____

14. Cite the other name for a hallux valgus.

_____

15. Name the injury that involves the semilunar cartilages in the knee.

_____

16. List the three abnormal curvatures of the spine.

_____

17. Identify the structures in the skeletal system affected by osteoarthritis.

_____

_____

18. What year was Lyme disease first detected?

_____

19. List the classic symptoms of bursitis.

_____

_____

20. Name the medication that may be injected into the joint to treat bursitis.

_____

21. Identify the area of the foot that is usually affected by gout.

_____

22. Is Ewing's sarcoma encapsulated?

_____

23. What determines the prognosis for primary bone cancer?

_____

24. List the terms used to classify sprains.

_____

25. Gangrene, severe trauma, malignancy, or congenital defects are some conditions that may necessitate surgical removal of a limb. Name the procedure.

_____

26. Are muscle tumors often benign?

_____

27. Which area of the body is affected when a person has plantar fasciitis?

_____

28. What can a person do to prevent heel spurs?

_____

FILL IN THE BLANKS

Fill in the blanks with the correct terms. A word list has been provided. Words used twice are indicated with a (2).

1. All movement, including the movement of the _____ themselves and of the _____ is performed by _____ tissue.

2. The three types of muscle tissue are _____ or skeletal, _____ or smooth, and _____.

3. Bones develop through a process called _____.

4. The complete skeleton is formed by the end of the _____ month of _____.

5. Joints are classified according to their _____.

6. _____ is a semismooth, dense, supporting connective _____ that is found at the _____ of _____.

7. A patient with fibromyalgia has a relatively low level of the brain nerve chemical _____.

8. Bursae are found between _____ and _____ and cover _____ prominences, _____ movement.

9. The most commonly involved bones in osteomyelitic infections are the upper ends of the _____ and _____, the lower end of the _____, and occasionally the _____.

10. Phantom _____ sensation is an unpleasant complication that sometimes follows a(an) _____.

11. Permanent _____ can result from tendon damage.

12. A _____ most commonly develops on the _____ of the wrist as a single, _____ lump, just under the _____ of the skin.

WORD LIST

amputation, back, body, bones, bony, cardiac, cartilage, ends, facilitating, femur, ganglion, gestation, humerus, limb, movement, muscle, muscle atrophy, muscles, nonstriated, organs, osteogenesis, serotonin, smooth, striated, surface, tendons, third, tibia, tissue, vertebrae

ANATOMIC STRUCTURES

Identify the structures of the following anatomic diagrams.

1. Normal muscular system—anterior view

(1) _____   (8) _____

(2) _____   (9) _____

(3) _____   (10) _____

(4) _____   (11) _____

(5) _____   (12) _____

(6) _____   (13) _____

(7) _____   (14) _____

2. Normal muscular system—posterior view

(1) _____   (6) _____

(2) _____   (7) _____

(3) _____   (8) _____

(4) _____   (9) _____

(5) _____

3. Types of muscles

_____

_____

_____

4. Normal skeletal system—anterior view

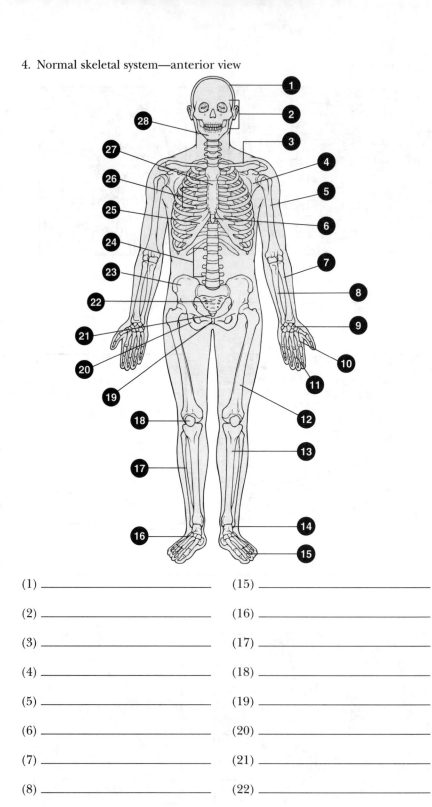

(1) _____   (15) _____

(2) _____   (16) _____

(3) _____   (17) _____

(4) _____   (18) _____

(5) _____   (19) _____

(6) _____   (20) _____

(7) _____   (21) _____

(8) _____   (22) _____

(9) _____   (23) _____

(10) _____   (24) _____

(11) _____   (25) _____

(12) _____   (26) _____

(13) _____   (27) _____

(14) _____   (28) _____

5. Examples of types of joints

_____

_____

_____

_____

_____

_____

_____

_____

6. Types of fractures

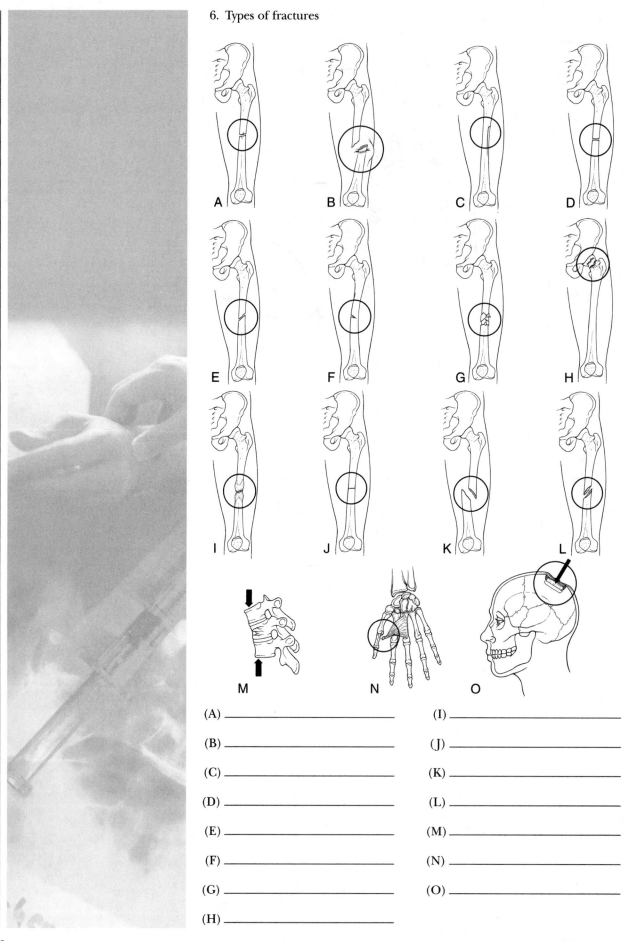

(A) _____

(B) _____

(C) _____

(D) _____

(E) _____

(F) _____

(G) _____

(H) _____

(I) _____

(J) _____

(K) _____

(L) _____

(M) _____

(N) _____

(O) _____

PATIENT SCREENING

For each scenario that follows, explain how and why you would schedule an appointment or suggest a referral based on the patient's reported symptoms. First, review the "Guidelines for Patient Screening Exercises" found on page iii in the "Introduction."

1. The mother of a 12-year-old girl calls in saying her daughter has started complaining of back pain and fatigue. She also states that she has noticed her daughter's skirts do not hang evenly and that the school nurse has suggested an examination for scoliosis. How do you handle this phone call?

   _____

   _____

   _____

2. A patient calls in asking for an appointment saying that he has a red, itchy rash with a red circle center resembling the bull's eye on a target (target lesion) on his arm. He tells you he was out in the woods 2 days ago and thinks that a tick bit him. He thinks that the physician should see him. How do you respond to this call?

   _____

   _____

   _____

3. A male patient calls in telling you that he is experiencing severe, almost excruciating pain in the first joint of his left great toe. He has experienced this before and the pain usually will peak after several hours and then subside gradually. He also has a slight fever and chills. How do you respond to this call?

   _____

   _____

   _____

4. A patient calls the office saying he just twisted his ankle while walking up the stairs. He is complaining of localized pain and says he cannot stand on his leg. How do you handle this call?

   _____

   _____

   _____

5. A patient calls in saying while she was cutting a watermelon her knife slipped and she cut the middle finger on her left hand. The bleeding is controlled but she cannot bend her finger. The physician is gone from the office for the day. How do you handle this call?

   _____

   _____

PATIENT TEACHING

For each scenario below, outline the appropriate patient teaching you would perform. First, review the "Guidelines for Patient-Teaching Exercises" found on page iv in the "Introduction."

1. OSTEOARTHRITIS

   An established patient with a history of osteoarthritis is undergoing on-going therapy, which includes drug therapy and a gentle exercise regimen. The patient is discouraged because of increased pain and loss of mobility. The physician instructs you to provide printed information regarding therapeutic diets and exercise for the patient. Additionally, you are to review intended effects of the prescribed drug therapy. How do you handle this patient-teaching opportunity?

   _____

   _____

   _____

   _____

2. LYME DISEASE

   A male patient has been diagnosed with Lyme disease. Antibiotic therapy has been prescribed. The patient has been told to return for a checkup in 1 week. The physician asks you to provide the patient with printed information concerning therapy that is advised in the treatment of this condition. How would you handle this patient-teaching opportunity?

   _____

   _____

   _____

   _____

   _____

3. GOUT

   An individual has been diagnosed with gout. The physician has instructed you to provide the patient with printed information regarding therapy for treatment of gout. How do you approach this patient-teaching opportunity?

   _____

   _____

   _____

   _____

4. OSTEOPOROSIS

An older woman has been diagnosed with osteoporosis. The physician asks you to provide the patient with printed information concerning therapy that is advised in the treatment of this condition. How do you handle this patient-teaching opportunity?

_____

_____

_____

_____

5. FRACTURES

An individual has a fracture of the ulna and radius at the wrist. A cast was placed on the area a few weeks earlier, and the patient is now requesting additional information about therapy for the hand, wrist, and arm. The physician has explained the anticipated therapy to the patient and requests you review this information with him or her. How do you handle this patient-teaching opportunity?

_____

_____

_____

_____

PHARMACOLOGY QUESTIONS

Circle the letter of the choice that best completes the statement or answers the question.

1. Which of the following medications is classified as a muscle relaxant?
   a. Celecoxib (Celebrex)
   b. Ibuprofen (Motrin)
   c. Cyclobenzaprine (Flexeril)
   d. Colchicine

2. Treatment of fibromyalgia may include all of the following except
   a. Naproxen (Naprosyn)
   b. Amitriptyline (Elavil)
   c. Alendronate (Fosamax)
   d. Oxaprozin (Daypro)

3. Which of the following antiinflammatory drugs has been reported to have less GI irritation?
   a. Indomethacin (Indocin)
   b. Celecoxib (Celebrex)
   c. Naproxen (Naprosyn)
   d. Oxaprozin (Daypro)

4. Bursitis is commonly treated with the following, except for
   a. Application of moist heat.
   b. Nonsteroidal antiinflammatory drugs.
   c. Corticosteroid drugs.
   d. Muscle relaxants.

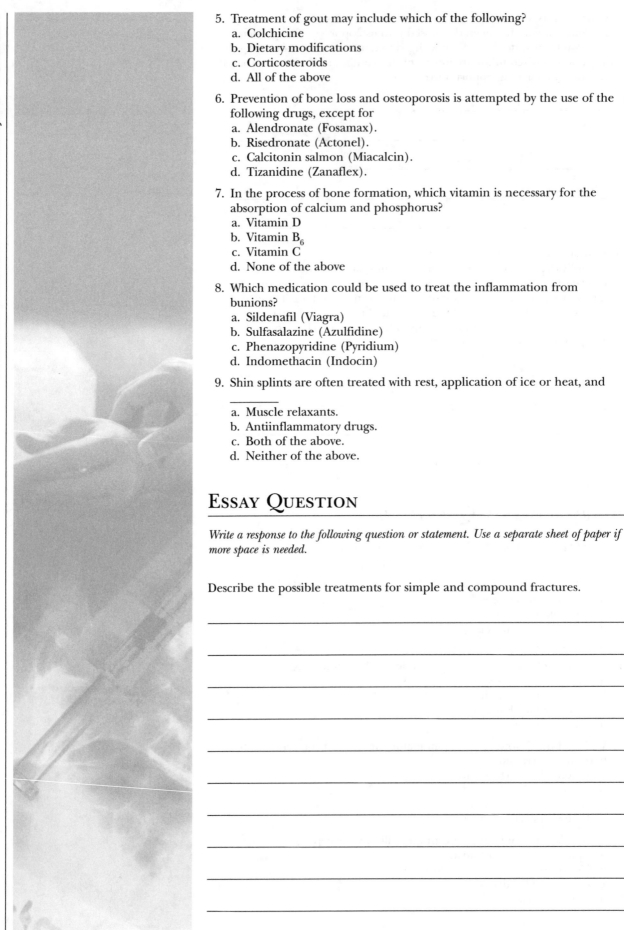

5. Treatment of gout may include which of the following?
   a. Colchicine
   b. Dietary modifications
   c. Corticosteroids
   d. All of the above

6. Prevention of bone loss and osteoporosis is attempted by the use of the following drugs, except for
   a. Alendronate (Fosamax).
   b. Risedronate (Actonel).
   c. Calcitonin salmon (Miacalcin).
   d. Tizanidine (Zanaflex).

7. In the process of bone formation, which vitamin is necessary for the absorption of calcium and phosphorus?
   a. Vitamin D
   b. Vitamin B_6
   c. Vitamin C
   d. None of the above

8. Which medication could be used to treat the inflammation from bunions?
   a. Sildenafil (Viagra)
   b. Sulfasalazine (Azulfidine)
   c. Phenazopyridine (Pyridium)
   d. Indomethacin (Indocin)

9. Shin splints are often treated with rest, application of ice or heat, and _____
   a. Muscle relaxants.
   b. Antiinflammatory drugs.
   c. Both of the above.
   d. Neither of the above.

ESSAY QUESTION

Write a response to the following question or statement. Use a separate sheet of paper if more space is needed.

Describe the possible treatments for simple and compound fractures.

_____

_____

_____

_____

_____

_____

_____

_____

CERTIFICATION EXAMINATION REVIEW

Circle the letter of the choice that best completes the statement or answers the question.

1. Lordosis is a(an) _____ curvature of the spine.
   a. Lateral
   b. Inward (swayback)
   c. Outward
   d. None of the above

2. Scoliosis is a(an) _____ curvature of the spine.
   a. Lateral
   b. Inward (swayback)
   c. Outward
   d. None of the above

3. Kyphosis is a(an) _____ curvature of the spine.
   a. Lateral
   b. Inward (swayback)
   c. Outward
   d. None of the above

4. Gouty arthritis is an inflammation of the joints caused by
   a. An excessive level of uric acid in the joints.
   b. An excessive level of serum protein.
   c. Streptococcus bacteria.
   d. None of the above.

5. A fracture with a break in the bone and a wound is a _____ fracture.
   a. Spiral
   b. Comminuted
   c. Compound, through the skin
   d. None of the above

6. A fracture with splintered or crushed bone is a
   a. Comminuted fracture
   b. Simple fracture
   c. Greenstick fracture
   d. None of the above

7. When a bone is fractured as a result of disease, it is called a _____ fracture.
   a. Greenstick
   b. Pathologic
   c. Spiral fracture
   d. None of the above

8. Atrophy is the wasting away or deterioration of a
   a. Bone.
   b. Ligament.
   c. Muscle.
   d. None of the above.

9. A severed tendon causes immediate and severe pain, inflammation, and
   a. Decreases mobility of the affected part.
   b. Complete immobility of the affected part.
   c. Weakness of the affected part.
   d. None of the above.

10. Spurs are a common problem diagnosed in
    a. Individuals with bone deficiency.
    b. Individuals active in sports, especially runners.
    c. Individuals who use repetitive hand and wrist motions in their employment.
    d. None of the above.

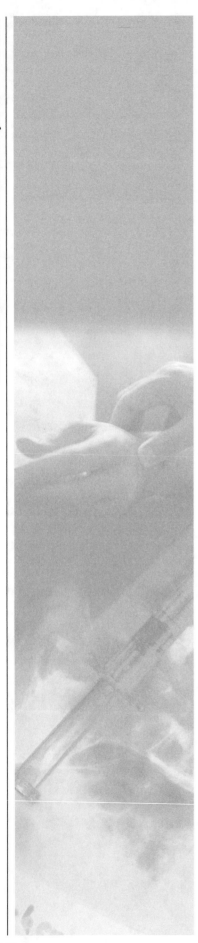

11. Lyme disease is transmitted from a bacteria that is carried by a
    a. Mosquito.
    b. Bee.
    c. Tick.
    d. All of the above.

12. Tendons are tough strands or cords of dense connective tissue that attach muscle to
    a. Muscle.
    b. Joints.
    c. Bones.
    d. None of the above.

13. Collagen is a major supporting element or glue in
    a. Muscles.
    b. Ligaments.
    c. Connective tissue.
    d. None of the above.

14. The skeletal system is composed of _____ bones.
    a. 200
    b. 208
    c. 308
    d. None of the above

15. Osteomyelitis is a(an)
    a. Chronic progressive inflammatory disease.
    b. Infection in a bone that can lead to abscess formation and sequestrum when not properly cared for.
    c. Progressive weakening of the skeletal muscles.
    d. None of the above.

16. Adhesive capsulitis (frozen shoulder)
    a. Can result in permanent impairment of mobility of the shoulder.
    b. Occurs more frequently in patients with diabetes.
    c. Usually begins after an injury, or a case of bursitis or tendinitis.
    d. All of the above.

17. Symptoms and signs of bone tumors may include
    a. Pain.
    b. No pain.
    c. A limp.
    d. All of the above.

CHAPTER 8

Diseases and Conditions of the Digestive System

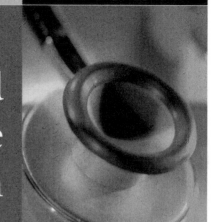

WORD DEFINITIONS

Define the following basic medical terms:

1. Apicectomy   _____

2. Cholinergic   _____

3. Colectomy   _____

4. Erosion   _____

5. Fissure   _____

6. Fistula   _____

7. Gangrene   _____

8. Hematemesis   _____

9. Leukoplakia   _____

10. Ligation   _____

11. Lymphadenopathy   _____

12. Malaise   _____

13. Metastasis   _____

14. Odynophagia   _____

15. Pseudomembranous   _____

16. Retrosternal   _____

17. Valsalva's maneuver   _____

GLOSSARY TERMS

Define the following chapter glossary terms:

1. Anastomoses _____
2. Aphthous ulcers _____
3. Cachexia _____
4. Diaphoretic _____
5. Fissures _____
6. Fistulas _____
7. Gangrene _____
8. H$_2$-receptor antagonist _____
9. Hemostasis _____
10. Hepatomegaly _____
11. Hyperemic _____
12. Hypovolemic shock _____
13. Jaundiced _____
14. Lavage _____
15. Malocclusion _____
16. Myalgia _____
17. Peritonitis _____
18. Proton pump inhibitor _____
19. Reflux _____
20. Steatorrhea _____

SHORT ANSWER

Answer the following questions:

1. Identify the function of the teeth.

   _____

2. List three reasons that a person may be missing permanent teeth.

   _____

   _____

3. Describe how oral tumors begin.

_____

4. What symptom usually prompts a person to seek medical treatment for temporomandibular joint syndrome?

_____

5. Is thrush a bacterial, fungal, or viral infection?

_____

6. Cite statistics of incidence of squamous cell oral cancers.

_____

7. What lifestyle factors contribute to up to 80% of cases of oral cancer?

_____

_____

8. List treatment options for oral cancer.

_____

_____

9. Identify the main symptom that a patient experiences with esophagitis.

_____

10. Name the main cause of gastritis.

_____

11. Name the country with the highest incidence of gastric cancer in the world.

_____

12. What condition is considered the main risk factor for development of gastric cancer in the proximal stomach?

_____

13. Cite the length of the appendix.

_____

14. Identify the function of the appendix.

_____

15. Name the device that patients sometimes wear if they have a hernia.

_____

16. Identify the area of the alimentary canal that can be affected by Crohn's disease.

_____

17. Name the type of cancer that a patient with chronic ulcerative colitis is at risk to develop.

_____

18. Explain the goal of treatment for gastroenteritis.

_____

_____

19. List the symptoms and signs of intestinal obstruction.

_____

20. Which portion of the colon is usually the site of diverticulosis?

_____

21. Name the third most common site of cancer incidence and cause of death in both men and women.

_____

22. At what age should annual fecal occult testing begin for people at average risk for colorectal cancer?

_____

23. Can peritonitis be life threatening?

_____

24. In which sex is cirrhosis diagnosed more frequently?

_____

25. Identify the incubation period for hepatitis A.

_____

26. List the four fat-soluble vitamins that are stored in fat tissue.

_____

FILL IN THE BLANKS

Fill in the blanks with the correct terms. A word list has been provided. Words used twice are indicated with a (2).

1. The _____ processes and transports products of

_____.

2. The function of the teeth is _____ to break down food

into pieces that can be _____ and digested

_____.

3. Periodontitis, also called _____ disease, is destructive

_____ and bone _____ around one or

more of the _____.

4. A _____ is a pus-filled sac that develops in the

_____ surrounding the _____ of the root.

5. Herpes simplex blisters can develop on the _____ and

inside the _____, producing painful _____

that last a few hours or _____.

6. Oral cancer usually appears as a _____, patchy lesion or

an _____ ulcer that _____ to heal.

7. Normal esophageal reflux can result from _____,

pregnancy, or _____ gain.

8. Treatment of esophagitis includes several weeks of a

_____ to calm the _____ and the use of

_____ antacids.

9. A _____ hernia exists when the _____

part of the _____ protrudes through the

_____ opening of the diaphragm into the thoracic cavity.

10. A _____ is a mechanical bowel obstruction where there is

a twisting of the bowel on itself.

11. Short-bowel _____ is the result of an

_____ amount of functioning small bowel to

_____ nutrients, fluid, _____, and

minerals that the body needs.

12. Hemorrhoids are _____ dilations of a vein in the

_____ or the anorectal area.

13. Viral hepatitis is _____ until _____ is

complete.

14. Celiac disease is a disease of the _____ that is

characterized by _____, _____, and

_____ to the lining of the intestine.

WORD LIST

absorb, alimentary canal, anal canal, base, bland diet, bone, contagious, damage, days, digestion, easily, esophageal, fails, gluten intolerance, gum, hiatal, inflammation, insufficient, lips, malabsorption, mastication, mouth, oral, overeating, periodontal, recovery, small intestine, stomach, strong, swallowed, syndrome, teeth, tissue, tooth abscess, ulcers, upper, varicose, vitamins, volvulus, weight, white

ANATOMIC STRUCTURES

Identify the following structures of the digestive system and their functions.

1. Main and accessory organs of the normal digestive system

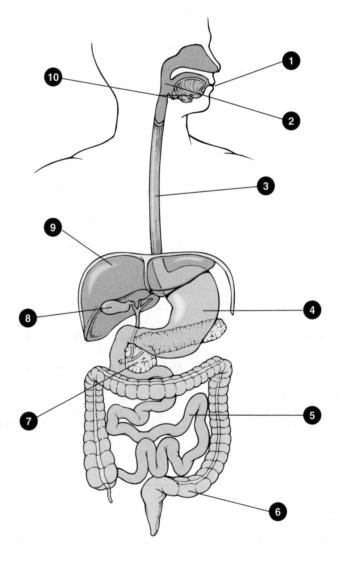

(1) _____

(2) _____

(3) _____

(4) _____

(5) _____

(6) _____

(7) _____

(8) _____

(9) _____

(10) _____

PATIENT SCREENING

For each scenario below, explain how and why you would schedule an appointment or suggest a referral based on the patient's reported symptoms. First, review the "Guidelines for Patient-Screening Exercises" found on page iii in the "Introduction."

1. A male patient calls stating he is experiencing pain in the "jaw joint" on the right side of his mouth. He says he has been hearing a clicking sound when he chews and the pain is getting progressively worse. He also says he is having problems opening his mouth. He requests an appointment to see the physician. How do you handle this phone call?

   _____

   _____

   _____

2. A patient calls stating he is experiencing "heartburn," usually most severe at night. He also says he has episodes of belching, causing a burning sensation in his mouth and chest. How do you handle this phone call?

   _____

   _____

   _____

3. The father of a 16-year-old adolescent calls the office stating his son is experiencing abdominal pain that started as vague discomfort around the navel. Now a few hours later, it has localized in the right lower quadrant. He has just become nauseated and has a slight fever. How do you handle this call?

   _____

   _____

   _____

4. A patient calls stating she is experiencing pain in the right upper quadrant of the abdomen, often radiating to the right upper back in the area of the scapula. Nausea and vomiting accompany the pain. She thinks her skin is turning yellow. How do you respond to this call?

_____

_____

_____

5. The mother of a 16-year-old adolescent calls in advising she wants her daughter to be seen by the physician. The girl is refusing to eat and is preoccupied with obesity and obsessed with her weight. Although she experiences continued weight loss, she does not believe anything is wrong. How do you handle this phone call?

_____

_____

_____

PATIENT TEACHING

For each scenario below, outline the appropriate patient teaching you would perform. First, review the "Guidelines for Patient-Teaching Exercises" found on page iv in the "Introduction."

1. DENTAL CARIES
   A patient is noted to be in need of dental assessment. The physician suggests that until a dental appointment can be made and kept, the patient should be instructed on proper oral hygiene and dental care. How do you handle this patient-teaching opportunity?

   _____

   _____

   _____

2. HERPES SIMPLEX
   A patient has a large "cold sore" on the upper lip that is quite painful. It is diagnosed as a herpes simplex eruption. You are instructed to provide printed information regarding the care of the eruption and ways to prevent spreading this contagious lesion. How do you approach this patient-teaching opportunity?

   _____

   _____

   _____

   _____

   _____

3. GASTROESOPHAGEAL REFLUX DISORDER

An individual experiencing gastroesophageal reflux disorder (GERD) requires instructions about methods to prevent the reflux. The physician requests you to provide him or her with printed information and to explain how he or she can lessen the occurrence of the attacks. How do you approach this patient-teaching opportunity?

_____

_____

_____

_____

_____

4. PEPTIC ULCERS

An individual has been diagnosed with a peptic ulcer. The physician requests that you reinforce his instructions to the patient by using printed material available in the office. How do you approach this patient-teaching opportunity?

_____

_____

_____

_____

_____

5. CHOLECYSTITIS

An individual has been experiencing severe right-sided epigastric pain after eating. The diagnosis of cholecystitis has been made. The physician requests you reinforce her dietary instructions to the patient using printed dietary information available in the office. How do you approach this patient-teaching opportunity?

_____

_____

_____

_____

_____

PHARMACOLOGY QUESTIONS

Circle the letter of the choice that best completes the statement or answers the question.

1. Some medications may cause discoloration of the teeth. Which of the following drugs has been shown to discolor teeth when taken during early childhood?
   a. Penicillin
   b. Sulfamethoxazole
   c. Tetracycline
   d. Prednisone

2. In advanced cases of gingivitis, which antibacterial mouthwash is frequently prescribed?
   a. Lugol's solution
   b. Listerine
   c. 0.9% sodium chloride
   d. Chlorhexidine (Periogard)

3. Oral thrush (*Candida albicans*) is often treated with which oral antifungal agent?
   a. Cephalexin (Keflex)
   b. Atorvastatin (Lipitor)
   c. Nystatin
   d. Simvastatin (Zocor)

4. Gastroesophageal reflux disease (GERD) may be treated with all of the following, except _____.
   a. Theophylline
   b. Omeprazole (Prilosec)
   c. A decrease in cigarette smoking
   d. Elevation of the head of the bed

5. Which of the following drugs should be avoided in a patient with peptic ulcer?
   a. Esomeprazole (Nexium)
   b. Naproxen sodium (Aleve)
   c. Ranitidine (Zantac)
   d. Cimetidine (Tagamet)

6. Which of the following is used to treat peptic ulcers?
   a. Lansoprazole (Prevacid)
   b. Pregabalin (Lyrica)
   c. Metformin (Glucophage)
   d. Glimepiride (Amaryl)

7. The treatment of ulcerative colitis may include all of the following, except _____?
   a. Corticosteroids
   b. Sulfasalazine (Azulfidine)
   c. Timolol (Timoptic)
   d. Anticholinergic agents

8. Inflammation of the peritoneum (peritonitis) may be treated with any or all of the following, except _____.
   a. Methylphenidate (Ritalin)
   b. Broad spectrum antibiotics
   c. Parenteral electrolytes
   d. Pain killers

9. Which of the following medications may be used to treat motion sickness?
   a. Cimetidine (Tagamet)
   b. Dimenhydrinate (Dramamine)
   c. Metoclopramide (Reglan)
   d. Omeprazole (Prilosec)

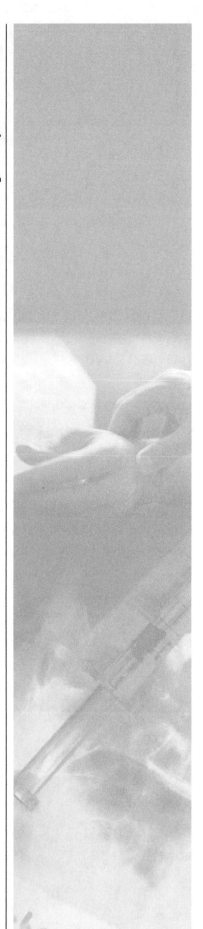

ESSAY QUESTION

Write a response to the following question or statement. Use a separate sheet of paper if more space is needed.

Describe the signs and symptoms that are associated with Crohn's disease and available options for treatment.

_____

_____

_____

_____

_____

_____

_____

_____

_____

CERTIFICATION EXAMINATION REVIEW

Circle the letter of the choice that best completes the statement or answers the question.

1. The transmission route for _____ is fecal oral and is transmitted by contaminated water, food, and stools. Poor hygiene also plays a role in the transmission.
   a. Hepatitis A
   b. Hepatitis B
   c. Hepatitis C
   d. None of the above

2. The use of broad-spectrum antibiotics is associated with the occurrence of
   a. Esophagitis.
   b. Gastritis.
   c. Pseudomembranous enterocolitis.
   d. None of the above.

3. The symptoms of biliary colic with radiating pain and jaundice accompany
   a. Appendicitis.
   b. Cholecystitis.
   c. Cholelithiasis.
   d. Both b and c.

4. Anorexia nervosa is an eating disorder in which the person perceives their body image as
   a. Thin.
   b. Just right.
   c. Overweight.
   d. None of the above.

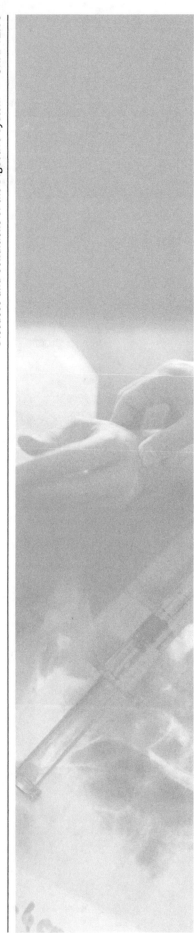

5. A chronic irreversible degeneration of the liver is
   a. Cholecystitis.
   b. Pancreatitis.
   c. Cholelithiasis.
   d. Cirrhosis.

6. The route of transmission for _____ is by blood or body fluid.
   a. Hepatitis A
   b. Hepatitis B
   c. Hepatitis C
   d. Both b and c

7. Peritonitis is an infection that involves the
   a. Liver.
   b. Serous membrane that lines the abdominal cavity.
   c. Pancreas.
   d. None of the above.

8. Neoplasm, volvulus, intussusception, and fecal impaction can all cause
   a. Diverticulitis.
   b. Diverticulosis.
   c. Mechanical bowel obstruction.
   d. None of the above.

9. The fourth leading cause of cancer-related death in the United States is
   a. Colon cancer.
   b. Gastric cancer.
   c. Pancreatic cancer.
   d. None of the above.

10. Allergic reaction or irritation from foods, mechanical injury, medications, poisons, alcohol, and infectious diseases may damage the gastric lining and cause
    a. Diverticulitis.
    b. Gastritis.
    c. Hepatitis.
    d. None of the above.

11. The following statements about periodontitis are true, except
    a. The cause is plaque biofilm.
    b. It is not related to gingivitis.
    c. Early detection and treatment can help prevent tooth loss.
    d. Chemotherapy, diabetes, smoking, and HIV are contributing factors.

12. The clinical management of Barrett's esophagus includes
    a. Treatment of the symptoms of GERD.
    b. Endoscopic surveillance every 3 years to detect dysplasia.
    c. Acid-suppressive medications, lifestyle changes, and possibly antireflux surgery.
    d. All of the above.

CHAPTER 9

Diseases and Conditions of the Respiratory System

Word Definitions

Define the following basic medical terms:

1. Auscultation _____

2. Dysphagia _____

3. Hepatomegaly _____

4. Hypercapnia _____

5. Hypocapnia _____

6. Laryngectomy _____

7. Mucopurulent _____

8. Myalgia _____

9. Opacities _____

10. Purulent _____

11. Rhinitis _____

12. Sclerosing _____

13. Suprasternal _____

14. Tinnitus _____

15. Venostasis _____

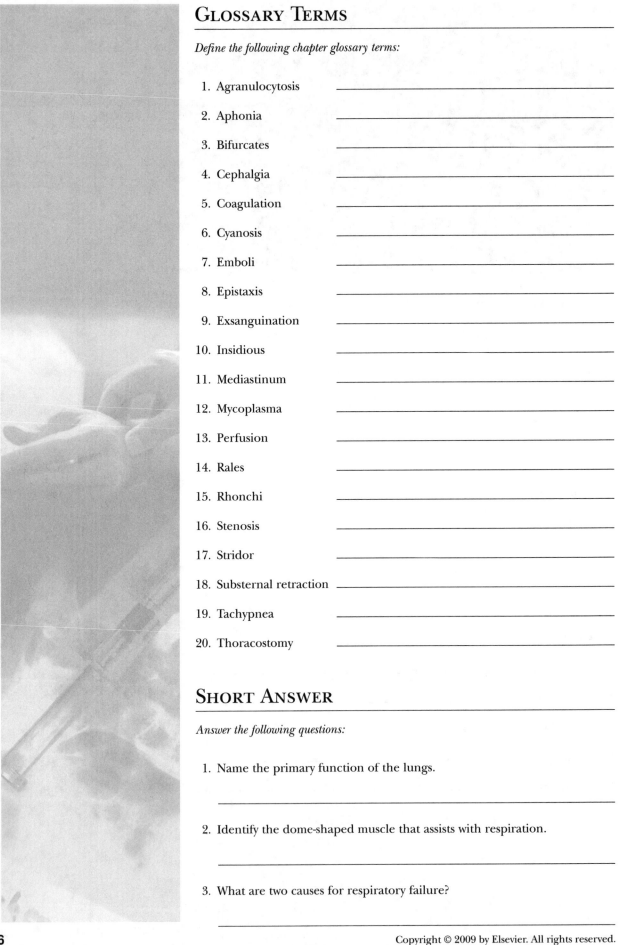

GLOSSARY TERMS

Define the following chapter glossary terms:

1. Agranulocytosis _____

2. Aphonia _____

3. Bifurcates _____

4. Cephalgia _____

5. Coagulation _____

6. Cyanosis _____

7. Emboli _____

8. Epistaxis _____

9. Exsanguination _____

10. Insidious _____

11. Mediastinum _____

12. Mycoplasma _____

13. Perfusion _____

14. Rales _____

15. Rhonchi _____

16. Stenosis _____

17. Stridor _____

18. Substernal retraction _____

19. Tachypnea _____

20. Thoracostomy _____

SHORT ANSWER

Answer the following questions:

1. Name the primary function of the lungs.

   _____

2. Identify the dome-shaped muscle that assists with respiration.

   _____

3. What are two causes for respiratory failure?

   _____

4. Does an antibiotic effectively treat a common cold?

_____

5. Identify the most common cause of sinusitis.

_____

6. What is the prognosis for emphysema?

_____

7. Name the most common symptom of nasopharyngeal carcinoma that is reported in over 90% of patients who are diagnosed with this type of cancer.

_____

8. What condition of the upper gastrointestinal (UGI) tract can result in laryngitis?

_____

9. Do nasal polyps tend to recur after surgical removal?

_____

10. When is a nosebleed considered an emergency?

_____

11. Identify the most common symptom of laryngeal neoplasms.

_____

12. Identify what occurs when a clot of foreign material lodges in and occludes an artery in the pulmonary circulation.

_____

13. Where do the vast majority of pulmonary emboli originate?

_____

14. Identify the age groups at most risk for respiratory syncytial viral (RSV) infection.

_____

15. Where is the causative agent of histoplasmosis found?

_____

16. What does the term pneumoconiosis mean?

_____

17. Name the condition that causes sharp needlelike pain and increases with inspiration and coughing.

_____

18. Identify the two types of pleurisy.

_____

19. What accumulates in the pleural cavity when hemothorax is the diagnosis?

_____

20. Describe the fracture that occurs when the patient is diagnosed with flail chest.

_____

21. Identify the intradermal test that is used to detect the presence of tuberculin antibodies.

_____

22. Is the prognosis for adult respiratory distress syndrome good or poor?

_____

23. Name the primary risk factor for developing lung cancer.

_____

24. What has contributed to the increase of tuberculosis in the United States?

_____

25. What patients are considered at high risk for aspiration pneumonia?

_____

FILL IN THE BLANKS

Fill in the blanks with the correct terms. A word list has been provided. Words used twice are indicated with a (2).

1. In the lungs, _____ inhaled from the air is

   _____ with _____ from the blood; this

   process is called _____ respiration.

2. On inspiration, the diaphragm _____, pulling downward

   and causing air to be _____ the lungs. During expiration,

   the diaphragm _____ pushing _____ and

   forcing air _____ of the lungs.

3. An ordinary cold should clear up in _____ to

   _____ days.

4. General _____ health _____ one to the

   common cold.

5. The sinuses, _____ in the bones lying

   _____ the nose, are normally _____ filled.

6. Because the opening of the larynx is _____, inflammation

   of the larynx sometimes _____ with _____.

7. Hemorrhage from the nose, known as _____, is a

   common _____ emergency.

8. The larynx plays an important role in _____, swallowing,

   _____, and protection of the _____

   airway.

9. Trauma, _____ of a _____, or

   _____ can cause bronchial bleeding, as can bronchitis or

   bronchiectasis.

10. Atelectasis follows incomplete _____ of the lobules or

    _____ of the _____, with partial or

    complete _____ of the lung.

11. Respiratory syncytial virus has the greatest occurrence during the

    _____ months.

12. Possible complications of influenza are _____, sinusitis,

    _____, and cervical _____.

13. Collapse of a lung causes severe _____ of

    _____, sudden sharp _____, falling

    _____, rapid _____ pulse, and

    _____ and weak _____.

14. The treatment for hemothorax includes reexpanding the lung, usually by

    _____ with closed _____ to evacuate the

    blood.

15. Pulmonary tuberculosis is acquired by the _____ of a

    _____ droplet _____ that contains the

    _____ _____.

WORD LIST

4, 5, air, behind, blood pressure, breath, breathing, bronchitis, calcification, carbon dioxide, cavities, chest pain, collapse, contracts, drainage, dried, epistaxis, erosion, exchanged, expansion, external, inhalation, interferes, lower, lungs, lymphadenopathy, narrow, nucleus, otitis media, out, oxygen, predisposes, poor, relaxes, respiration (2), segments, shallow, shortness, speech, sucked into, sudden, thoracostomy, tubercle bacillus, tumors, upward, vessel, weak, winter

ANATOMIC STRUCTURES

Identify the structures in the following anatomic diagrams.

1. Normal lower respiratory system

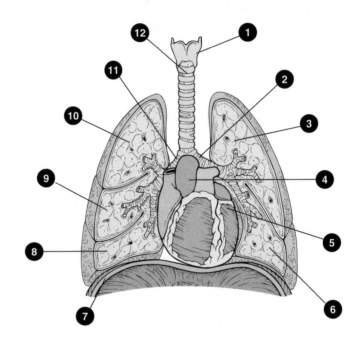

(1) _____   (7) _____

(2) _____   (8) _____

(3) _____   (9) _____

(4) _____   (10) _____

(5) _____   (11) _____

(6) _____   (12) _____

2. Normal upper respiratory system

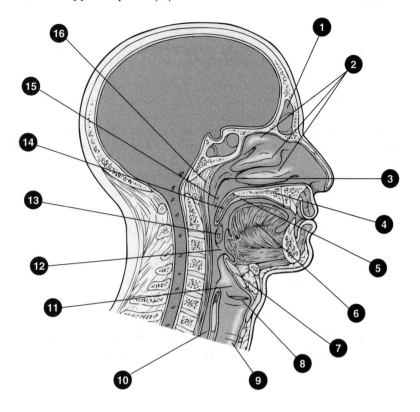

(1) _____

(2) _____

(3) _____

(4) _____

(5) _____

(6) _____

(7) _____

(8) _____

(9) _____

(10) _____

(11) _____

(12) _____

(13) _____

(14) _____

(15) _____

(16) _____

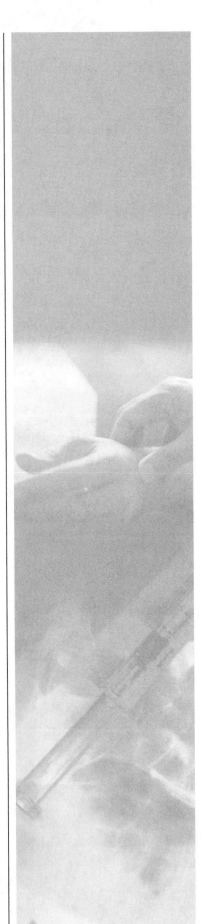

PATIENT SCREENING

For each scenario that follows, explain how and why you would schedule an appointment or suggest a referral based on the patient's reported symptoms. First, review the "Guidelines for Patient-Screening Exercises" found on page iii in the "Introduction."

1. A male patient calls in reporting he is experiencing headache over both eyes, especially on waking up in the morning. He also says there is pain and tenderness above the eyes, which occurs when bending over. Additionally, he reports a thick, greenish yellow drainage and has a slight temperature. How do you handle this phone call?

_____

_____

_____

_____

_____

2. A female patient calls in saying she is experiencing hoarseness, difficulty talking, a slight fever, and a sore throat. How do you respond to this call?

_____

_____

_____

_____

_____

3. A wife phones the office stating her husband is experiencing a severe nosebleed. The nose has been bleeding for about 20 minutes and they cannot get it to stop. How do you handle this phone call?

_____

_____

_____

_____

4. A male patient calls in saying he is coughing and spitting up blood. How do you respond to this call?

_____

_____

_____

_____

5. A female patient calls in and advises that she is experiencing a deep, persistent, productive cough. She has thick, yellow-to-gray sputum. Additionally, she reports shortness of breath, wheezing, a slightly elevated temperature, and pain in the upper chest, which is aggravated by the cough. How do you respond to this call?

_____

_____

_____

_____

_____

PATIENT TEACHING

For each scenario below, outline the appropriate patient teaching you would perform. First, review the "Guidelines for Patient-Teaching Exercises" found on page iv in the "Introduction."

1. PHARYNGITIS
   A patient has been diagnosed with recurrent pharyngitis. A course of antibiotic therapy has been prescribed. The physician has printed information regarding comfort measures. You are asked to provide the patient with the list, as well as encourage compliance with completing the antibiotic regimen. How do you approach this patient-teaching opportunity?

   _____

   _____

   _____

   _____

   _____

2. LARYNGITIS
   Recurring laryngitis has been diagnosed for a patient who can hardly speak. The physician instructs you to explain the importance of completing the antibiotic regimen. The office has printed instructions for the patient, and you are expected to provide the patient with the list and explain any areas not fully understood. How do you approach this patient-teaching opportunity?

   _____

   _____

   _____

   _____

   _____

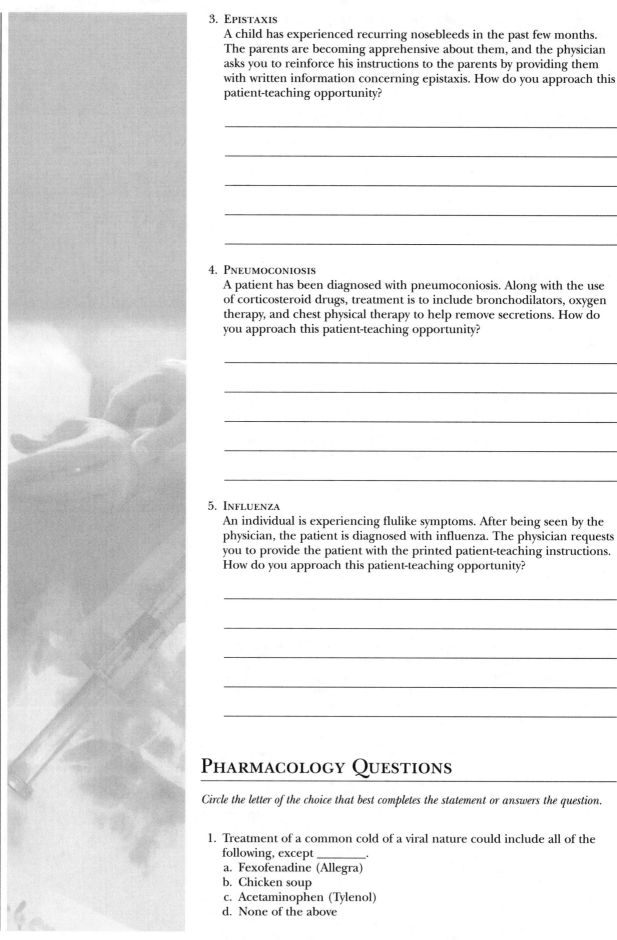

3. EPISTAXIS

A child has experienced recurring nosebleeds in the past few months. The parents are becoming apprehensive about them, and the physician asks you to reinforce his instructions to the parents by providing them with written information concerning epistaxis. How do you approach this patient-teaching opportunity?

_____

_____

_____

_____

_____

4. PNEUMOCONIOSIS

A patient has been diagnosed with pneumoconiosis. Along with the use of corticosteroid drugs, treatment is to include bronchodilators, oxygen therapy, and chest physical therapy to help remove secretions. How do you approach this patient-teaching opportunity?

_____

_____

_____

_____

_____

5. INFLUENZA

An individual is experiencing flulike symptoms. After being seen by the physician, the patient is diagnosed with influenza. The physician requests you to provide the patient with the printed patient-teaching instructions. How do you approach this patient-teaching opportunity?

_____

_____

_____

_____

_____

PHARMACOLOGY QUESTIONS

Circle the letter of the choice that best completes the statement or answers the question.

1. Treatment of a common cold of a viral nature could include all of the following, except _____.
   a. Fexofenadine (Allegra)
   b. Chicken soup
   c. Acetaminophen (Tylenol)
   d. None of the above

2. When sinusitis or pharyngitis is of a bacterial nature, which of the following would be considered proper treatment?
   a. Acyclovir (Zovirax)
   b. Oseltamivir (Tamiflu)
   c. Cephalexin (Keflex)
   d. None of the above

3. Treatment of pneumonia may include all of the following, except _____.
   a. Ciprofloxacin (Cipro)
   b. Tetracycline
   c. Acetaminophen (Tylenol)
   d. Dicyclomine (Bentyl)

4. Influenza can be treated with which of the following therapies?
   a. Bed rest
   b. Increased fluid intake
   c. Oseltamivir (Tamiflu)
   d. All of the above

5. Pulmonary emphysema can be treated with various therapies. Which of the following would not be a common treatment?
   a. Albuterol inhalation
   b. Ipratropium inhalation
   c. Furosemide (Lasix)
   d. Prednisone

6. Pleurisy is an inflammation of the membranes that surround the lungs. Which combination of medications would be the best therapy?
   a. Antibiotics and diuretics
   b. Antiinflammatories and beta blockers
   c. Antibiotics and beta blockers
   d. Antibiotics and analgesics

7. Infectious mononucleosis can be treated with all of the following therapies, except _____.
   a. Salmeterol inhaler (Serevent)
   b. Bed rest
   c. Adequate fluid intake
   d. Antipyretic medication

ESSAY QUESTION

Write a response to the following question or statement. Use a separate sheet of paper if more space is needed.

Discuss the importance of identifying patients with infectious tuberculosis, including measures of treatment.

_____

_____

_____

_____

_____

_____

_____

_____

_____

CERTIFICATION EXAMINATION REVIEW

Circle the letter of the choice that best completes the statement or answers the question.

1. Dysphonia is a common symptom of a
   a. Tumor of the bronchioles.
   b. Tumor of the lung.
   c. Tumor of larynx.
   d. None of the above.

2. Nasal polyps are growths that form from distended mucous membranes and protrude into the
   a. Sinus cavity.
   b. Throat.
   c. Nasal cavity.
   d. None of the above.

3. A pulmonary abscess is an area of contained _____ in the lung.
   a. Fluid
   b. Infectious material
   c. Tissue
   d. None of the above

4. Histoplasmosis is a _____ disease originating in the lungs with greatest occurrence in the Midwestern United States.
   a. Bacterial
   b. Fungal
   c. Viral
   d. None of the above

5. A pneumothorax is a collection of air or gas in the pleural cavity that can cause
   a. A collapsed lung.
   b. Lung cancer.
   c. A bacterial infection.
   d. All of the above.

6. Infectious mononucleosis is caused from
   a. Epstein-Barr virus.
   b. Histoplasmosis.
   c. Bacteria.
   d. None of the above.

7. Organism-specific antibiotics are used to treat
   a. Histoplasmosis.
   b. Mononucleosis.
   c. Bacterial pneumonia.
   d. All of the above.

8. Exposure to _____ smoke may make an individual more susceptible to any respiratory condition.
   a. Primary
   b. Secondary
   c. Both a and b
   d. None of the above

9. Pneumoconiosis is caused from inhalation of
   a. An airborne virus.
   b. Moisture droplets.
   c. Inorganic dust.
   d. All of the above.

10. Examples of occupational diseases include
    a. Pneumonia, sinusitis, and rhinitis.
    b. Asbestosis, anthracosis, and silicosis.
    c. Flail chest, pulmonary abscess, and emphysema.
    d. None of the above.

11. Legionellosis is a more severe form of Pontiac fever, and both forms are
    a. Contagious.
    b. Not contagious.
    c. Congenital.
    d. None of the above.

12. Barrel chest, chronic cough, and dyspnea are all symptoms of
    a. Emphysema.
    b. Pneumonia.
    c. Hemothorax.
    d. None of the above.

13. With flail chest, there are _____ fractures of three or more adjacent ribs.
    a. Single
    b. Double
    c. Both a and b
    d. Neither a or b

14. Sinusotomy, antibiotics, and decongestants may all be treatments for
    a. Sinusitis
    b. Bronchitis
    c. Allergic rhinitis
    d. None of the above

15. There are almost 200 different viruses that are responsible for causing
    a. Sinusitis.
    b. Bronchitis.
    c. The common cold.
    d. None of the above.

16. In the Southwest, coccidiomycosis is caused by a fungus, *Coccidioides immitis*. This is the agent that causes the disease known as
    a. Legionnaires' disease
    b. Histoplasmosis
    c. San Joaquin Valley Fever
    d. Asthma

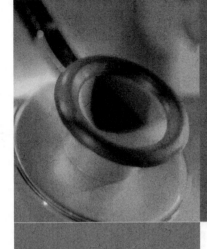

CHAPTER 10

Diseases and Conditions of the Circulatory System

WORD DEFINITIONS

Define the following basic medical terms:

1. Anticoagulant _____

2. Antipyretic _____

3. Arteritis _____

4. Atheroma _____

5. Bronchodilator _____

6. Carditis _____

7. Endocarditis _____

8. ESR _____

9. Gingival _____

10. Hyperlipidemia _____

11. Leukocytosis _____

12. Polyarthritis _____

13. Polycythemia _____

14. Serous _____

15. Transdermal _____

GLOSSARY TERMS

Define the following chapter glossary terms:

1. Aggregation   _____

2. Anaphylaxis   _____

3. Angina pectoris   _____

4. Angiotensin-
   converting enzyme   _____

5. Antibodies   _____

6. Arrhythmias   _____

7. Blood gas   _____

8. Bruit   _____

9. Collateral   _____

10. Commissurotomy   _____

11. Diuretics   _____

12. Doppler   _____

13. Gangrene   _____

14. Hematocrit   _____

15. Idiopathic   _____

16. Opacity   _____

17. Perfusion   _____

18. Petechiae   _____

19. Plaque   _____

20. Prophylactic   _____

21. Purpura   _____

22. Rales   _____

23. Sclerosing   _____

24. Syncope   _____

25. Tamponade   _____

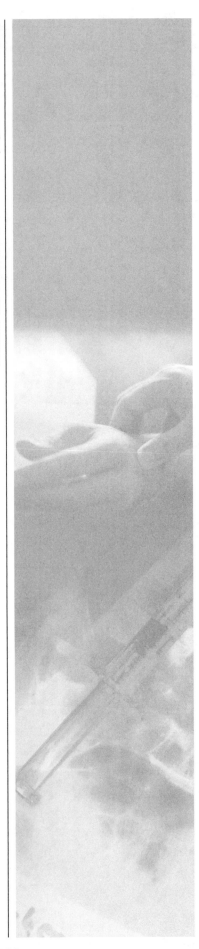

SHORT ANSWER

Answer the following questions:

1. The heart pumps how many quarts of blood throughout the body each minute?

   _____

2. Identify the first symptom of coronary artery disease.

   _____

3. List individuals having the potential to be at increased risk for coronary artery disease.

   _____

4. What is the term used to explain the new growth of blood vessels for patients with coronary artery disease (CAD)?

   _____

5. Describe the pain that is experienced by a patient experiencing angina pectoris.

   _____

6. Identify the forms of nitroglycerin that are helpful in preventing angina.

   _____

7. Cite the percentage of deaths occurring in the first hour after a myocardial infarction.

   _____

8. What measures are initiated to try to reverse cardiac arrest?

   _____

9. Name the most prevalent cardiovascular disorder in the United States.

   _____

10. List the symptoms of essential hypertension.

    _____

11. Are people always aware they have hypertension?

    _____

12. Identify the cardiac test that helps in evaluating cardiac chamber size, ventricular function, and disease of the myocardium, valves, cardiac strictures, and pericardium.

    _____

13. Cor pulmonale affects which side of the heart?

_____

14. Describe the skin of a person with pulmonary edema.

_____

15. What type of growths on the cardiac valves characterizes endocarditis?

_____

16. Identify a preventative measure before dental work for people with endocarditis.

_____

17. Which valves of the heart can be affected by valvular heart disease?

_____

18. Identify the cause of rheumatic heart disease.

_____

_____

19. Name the final option to treat rheumatic heart disease.

_____

20. List the symptoms associated with mitral valve prolapse.

_____

21. How are cardiac arrhythmias diagnosed?

_____

22. Which part of the heart fails to work effectively during cardiogenic shock?

_____

_____

23. Explain the cause of cardiac tamponade.

_____

24. List the three forms of arteriosclerosis.

_____

25. Which form of arteriosclerosis is responsible for most myocardial and cerebral infarctions?

_____

26. List the components of blood.

_____

27. What causes hemolytic anemia?

   _____

28. How are leukemias classified?

   _____

29. Name the form of leukemia that is the most common adult leukemia and accounts for 20% of childhood leukemias.

   _____

30. Identify the initial symptoms of Hodgkin's disease.

   _____

FILL IN THE BLANKS

Fill in the blanks with the correct terms. A word list has been provided. Words used twice are indicated with a (2).

1. The two upper chambers of the heart are called _____,

   _____, and the two lower chambers are called

   _____.

2. Cardiac muscle tissue is composed of _____

   _____ _____.

3. Myocardial infarction results from insufficient _____

   _____, as when a coronary _____ is

   occluded by atherosclerotic plaque, _____, or myocardial

   _____ spasm.

4. Cardiopulmonary resuscitation (CPR) must be instituted within

   _____ to _____ minutes of the

   _____ arrest.

5. Elevated _____ _____

   _____ are the _____ indication of

   hypertension.

6. Pulmonary edema causes patients to experience _____

   _____ and _____, orthopnea,

   _____ cardiac and respiratory _____, and

   often _____ frothy sputum.

7. Endocarditis is usually secondary to _____

_____ in the bloodstream.

8. Almost one third of all deaths in western countries are attributed to

_____ _____.

9. Deposits of fat-containing substances called _____

_____ on the _____ of the coronary

arteries result in atherosclerosis.

10. Angioplasty is attempted to open up a constricted _____

_____ in coronary artery disease.

11. Pulmonary edema is a condition of _____

_____ shift into the _____

_____ spaces of the lungs.

12. Cardiomyopathy causes the patient to experience symptoms of

_____ _____, including

_____ _____, _____,

_____, _____, and occasionally

_____ pain.

13. Myocarditis is frequently a _____, bacterial,

_____, or protozoal infection or complication of other

diseases.

14. Valvular heart disease can occur in the form of _____

_____ or _____ _____.

15. Arrhythmias occur when there is _____ with the

_____ system of the heart, resulting in an

_____ of the heartbeat.

WORD LIST

4, 6, abnormality, artery (2), atria, bacteria, blood pressure readings, bloody, cardiac, chest, congestive heart failure (CHF), conduction, coughing, dyspnea (2), extravascular, fatigue, first, fluid, fungal, heart disease, increased, insufficiency, interference, lumen, muscle, oxygen supply, palpitations, plaque, rates, stenosis, striated muscle cells, tachycardia, thrombus, ventricles, viral

ANATOMIC STRUCTURES

Identify the structures in the following anatomic diagrams. For number 4, identify what occurs with each phase of the cardiac cycle.

1. Anterior view of the heart and great vessels

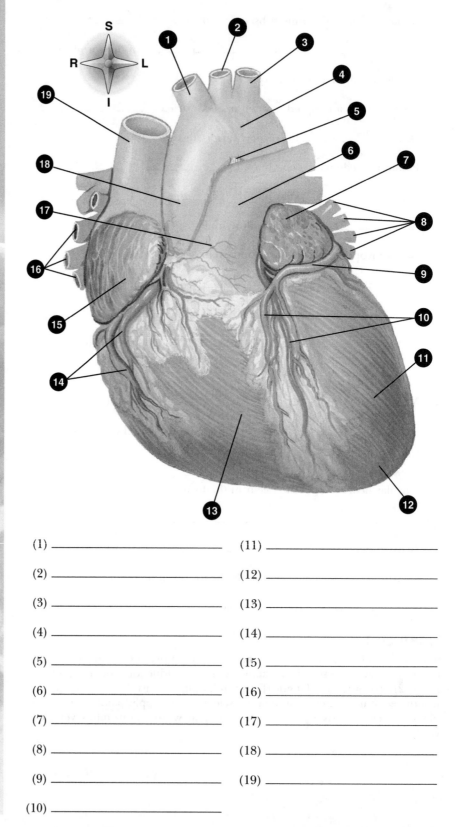

(1) _____   (11) _____

(2) _____   (12) _____

(3) _____   (13) _____

(4) _____   (14) _____

(5) _____   (15) _____

(6) _____   (16) _____

(7) _____   (17) _____

(8) _____   (18) _____

(9) _____   (19) _____

(10) _____

2. Posterior view of the heart and great vessels

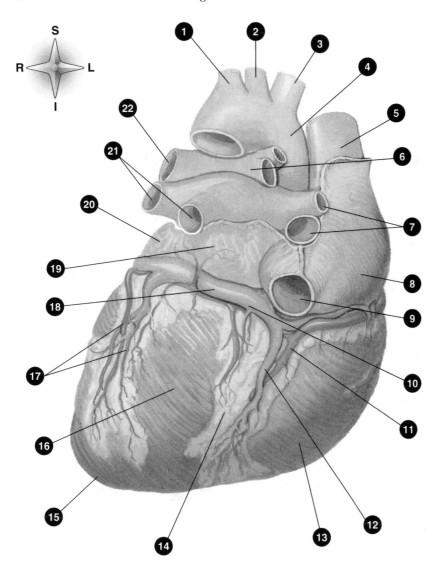

(1) _____

(2) _____

(3) _____

(4) _____

(5) _____

(6) _____

(7) _____

(8) _____

(9) _____

(10) _____

(11) _____

(12) _____

(13) _____

(14) _____

(15) _____

(16) _____

(17) _____

(18) _____

(19) _____

(20) _____

(21) _____

(22) _____

3. Circulation through the heart

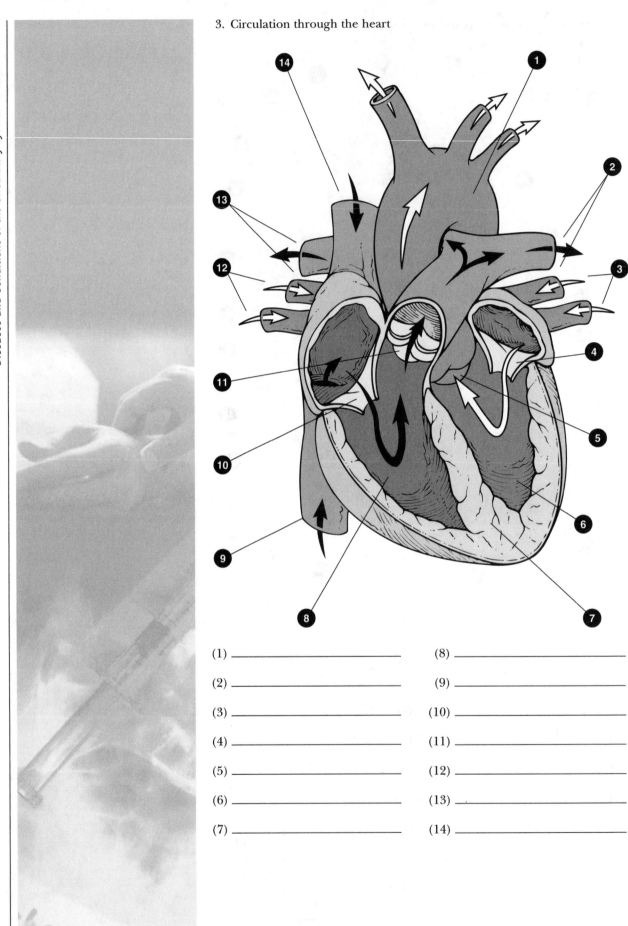

(1) _____	(8) _____
(2) _____	(9) _____
(3) _____	(10) _____
(4) _____	(11) _____
(5) _____	(12) _____
(6) _____	(13) _____
(7) _____	(14) _____

4. Cardiac cycle

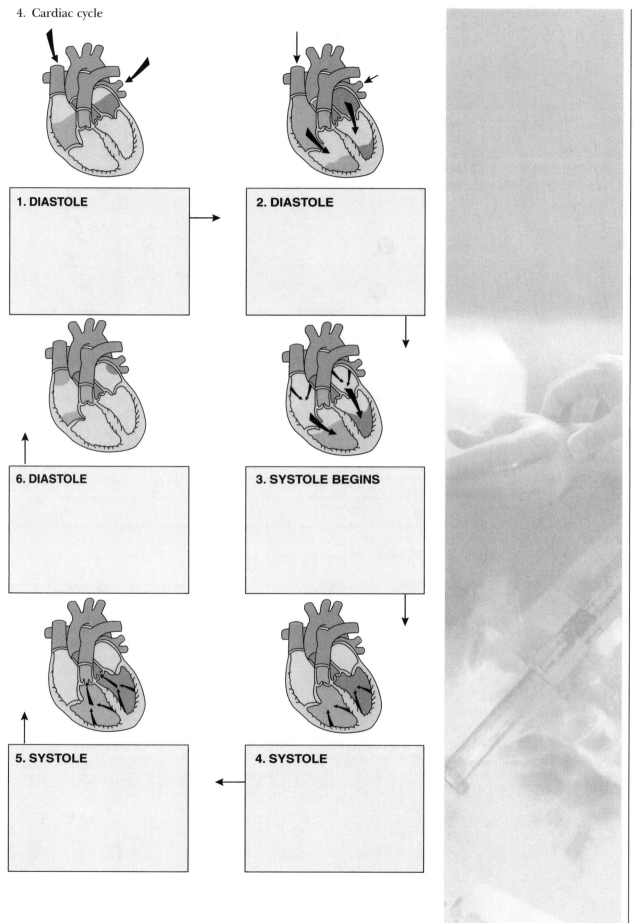

1. DIASTOLE

2. DIASTOLE

6. DIASTOLE

3. SYSTOLE BEGINS

5. SYSTOLE

4. SYSTOLE

5. Layers of the heart wall

(1) _____

(2) _____

(3) _____

(4) _____

(5) _____

(6) _____

(7) _____

6. Coronary arteries

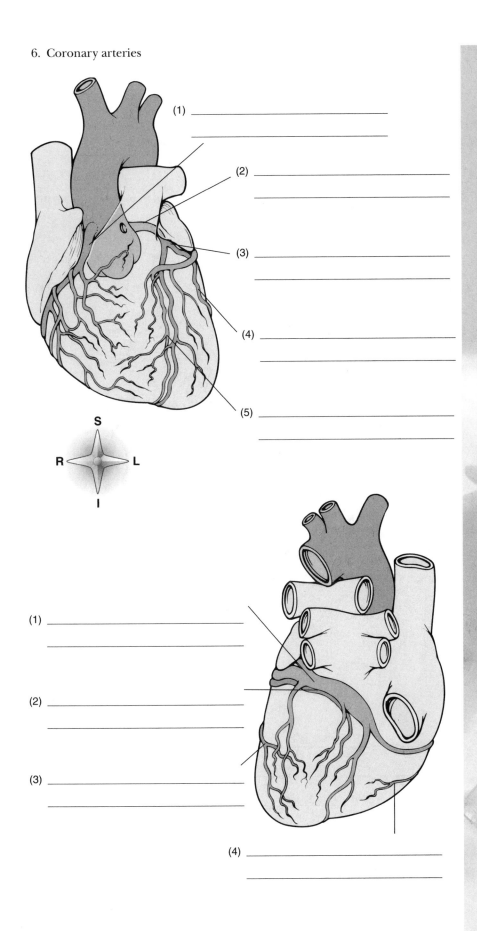

(1) _____

_____

(2) _____

_____

(3) _____

_____

(4) _____

_____

(5) _____

_____

(1) _____

_____

(2) _____

_____

(3) _____

_____

(4) _____

_____

7. Conduction system of the heart

(1) _____

(2) _____

(3) _____

(4) _____

(5) _____

(6) _____

PATIENT SCREENING

For each scenario that follows, explain how and why you would schedule an appointment or suggest a referral based on the patient's reported symptoms. First, review the "Guidelines for Patient-Screening Exercises" found on page iii in the "Introduction."

1. A patient's wife calls in stating her husband just experienced the sudden onset of left-sided chest pain after exertion. The pain has radiated to the left arm. The pain was relieved when he stopped the strenuous activity and placed a nitroglycerin tablet under his tongue. She wants to know if the physician should see him. How do you handle this call?

_____

_____

_____

_____

_____

_____

_____

2. A patient calls in saying she is experiencing headaches, light-headedness, and dizziness. She took her blood pressure at an automatic blood pressure screening station at the pharmacy, and the reading was 168/98. How do you handle this phone call?

_____

_____

_____

_____

_____

_____

_____

3. The husband of a patient calls in reporting his wife started having swollen feet and ankles, weight increase, and slight shortness of breath. She has a history of congestive heart failure. How do you handle this call?

_____

_____

_____

_____

_____

_____

_____

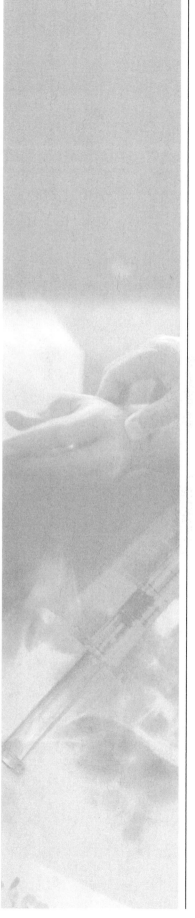

4. The patient calls in reporting pain and tenderness in the left leg that is becoming more severe. She has noted swelling, redness, warmth, and the development of a tender cordlike mass under the skin. How do you handle this call?

_____

_____

_____

_____

_____

5. The patient calls the office and says she is experiencing fatigue, and her skin—especially her hands—looks pale to her. She has had a few brief episodes of shortness of breath and a "pounding heart." How do you respond to this phone call?

_____

_____

_____

_____

_____

_____

Patient Teaching

For each scenario below, outline the appropriate patient teaching you would perform. First, review the "Guidelines for Patient-Teaching Exercises" found on page iv in the "Introduction."

1. Coronary artery disease (CAD)

A patient has recently been diagnosed with CAD. She has returned to the office for additional patient teaching concerning this condition. The office has printed material outlining emergency medical intervention in the event of chest pain, and the prevention and control of the disorder. The physician requests you provide this material to the patient and review it with her. How do you approach this patient-teaching opportunity?

_____

_____

_____

2. HYPERTENSION

A patient diagnosed with hypertension is in the office for a blood pressure recheck. He makes the statement that because his blood pressure is much better today, it will be possible to stop taking the medication. The physician requests that you reinforce his instructions that the medication still needs to be taken on a regular basis. The office has printed material available to give to hypertensive patients. How do you approach this patient-teaching opportunity?

_____

_____

_____

_____

3. CONGESTIVE HEART FAILURE (CHF)

A patient is experiencing recurring CHF. The physician requests you reinforce his instructions to the patient and the family regarding treatment of the condition. How do you approach this patient-teaching opportunity?

_____

_____

_____

_____

4. ATHEROSCLEROSIS

A diagnosis of atherosclerosis has been confirmed. The physician requests your assistance in reinforcing her recommendations to the patient. The office has printed materials regarding this condition and you are instructed to review these with the patient. How do you approach this patient-teaching opportunity?

_____

_____

_____

_____

5. RAYNAUD'S PHENOMENON

It is a very cold day, and the patient has just seen the physician after a severe attack of her condition. Even though the physician has previously advised her about the importance of avoiding situations where she is exposed to severe cold, she continues to go outside without gloves and head covering. The physician requests you provide the patient with printed information concerning her condition and reinforce the fact that exposure to severe cold will cause severe pain. How do you approach this patient-teaching opportunity?

_____

_____

_____

_____

PHARMACOLOGY QUESTIONS

Circle the letter of the choice that best completes the statement or answers the question.

1. Angina pectoris is commonly treated with sublingual nitroglycerin tablets. Which of the following is correct concerning the use of nitroglycerin?
   a. Sublingual tablets are kept in original glass container.
   b. Tablets should be kept in the refrigerator after opening.
   c. Sublingal tablets are explosive and should be handled carefully.
   d. None of the above.

2. Cardiac arrest is the sudden unexpected cessation of the heart. Which of the following interventions would be expected to be taken?
   a. Lidocaine injection
   b. CPR
   c. Sublingual beta adrenergic drugs
   d. a and b

3. Which of the following medications are not commonly used to treat hypertension?
   a. Candesartan (Atacand)
   b. Glyburide (Diabeta)
   c. Atenolol (Tenormin)
   d. Furosemide (Lasix)

4. Which of the following drugs should be avoided in a patient with hypertension?
   a. Hydrochlorothiazide
   b. Lisinopril (Zestril)
   c. Pseudoephedrine (Sudafed)
   d. Verapamil (Calan)

5. Congestive heart failure (CHF) is frequently treated with which of the following medications?
   a. Vasodilators
   b. Beta blockers
   c. Digoxin
   d. All of the above

6. The use of which of the following medicines is discouraged when a patient is taking nitrate based vasodilators?
   a. Hydrochlorothiazide
   b. Beta blockers
   c. Sildenafil (Viagra)
   d. Calcium channel blockers

7. Which of the following medications may be used in the treatment of cardiomyopathy?
   a. Digoxin (Lanoxin)
   b. Warfarin (Coumadin)
   c. Metformin (Glucophage)
   d. Both a and b

8. Medications used to treat endocarditis would most often include _____. (best answer)
   a. Antiinflammatories
   b. Antibiotics
   c. Antipyretics
   d. Antifungals

9. Which of the following drugs would be best at preventing thrombi?
   a. Digoxin (Lanoxin)
   b. Dicyclomine (Bentyl)
   c. Dexamethasone (Decadron)
   d. Warfarin (Coumadin)

10. Which of the following treatments would not be acceptable for the treatment of shock?
    a. Elevation of the legs
    b. IV fluid replacement
    c. Application of ice packs
    d. Maintain proper ventilation

11. Which of the following is not a drug used to treat elevated cholesterol levels?
    a. Simvastatin (Zocor)
    b. Ezetimibe (Zetia)
    c. Niacin
    d. Methylprednisolone (Medrol)

12. Which of the following statements is true?
    a. Heparin can be given orally or IV.
    b. Warfarin has a faster onset of action.
    c. Heparin is given by injection only.
    d. Warfarin comes in only one strength of tablet.

13. Which of the following medications are frequently used in the treatment of anemia?
    a. Vitamin D
    b. Iron
    c. Folic acid
    d. Vitamin B_{12} (cyanocobalamin)

ESSAY QUESTION

Write a response to the following question or statement. Use a separate sheet of paper if more space is needed.

Describe the laboratory tests that are used to confirm a diagnosis of acute lymphocytic leukemia (ALL).

_____

_____

_____

_____

_____

_____

_____

_____

_____

_____

_____

_____

_____

_____

_____

_____

_____

_____

_____

_____

_____

_____

_____

_____

_____

_____

_____

CERTIFICATION EXAMINATION REVIEW

Circle the letter of the choice that best completes the statement or answers the question.

1. A person who complains of experiencing chest pain with exertion is having
   a. Angina pectoris.
   b. A myocardial infarction.
   c. Shortness of breath.
   d. None of the above.

2. Pericarditis is an inflammation of the
   a. Myocardium.
   b. Endocardium.
   c. Sac enclosing the heart.
   d. None of the above.

3. Raynaud's disease is a vasospastic disease that affects the
   a. Heart.
   b. Legs and arms.
   c. Hands, fingers, and feet.
   d. None of the above.

4. The diagnosis of anemia indicates that the patient is experiencing a reduction in
   a. Red blood cells or hemoglobin.
   b. Platelets.
   c. Lymphatic tissue.
   d. None of the above.

5. The hereditary blood disease sickle cell anemia is predominantly seen in
    a. The white race.
    b. The black race.
    c. Both a and b.
    d. None of the above.

6. The lymphatic tissue in Hodgkin's disease patients contains
    a. Sickle cells.
    b. Monocytes.
    c. Reed-Sternberg cells.
    d. None of the above.

7. Rheumatic heart disease may cause problems with the
    a. Myocardium.
    b. Valves.
    c. Atria.
    d. None of the above.

8. Left-sided crushing-type chest pain, irregular heartbeat, dyspnea, and excessive sweating, nausea, anxiety, and denial are all symptoms of
    a. Mitral stenosis.
    b. Angina pectoris.
    c. Myocardial infarction.
    d. All of the above.

9. Electrocution, myocardial infarction, and drug overdose may cause
    a. Hypertension.
    b. Cardiac arrest.
    c. Cardiomyopathy.
    d. None of the above.

10. People with mitral valve prolapse are sometimes
    a. Asymptomatic.
    b. Anxious.
    c. Experiencing heart palpitations.
    d. All of the above.

11. Primary or essential hypertension
    a. Is related to lifestyle habits.
    b. Is genetic.
    c. Has an unknown etiology.
    d. None of the above.

12. Ischemia causes
    a. Death to tissue.
    b. Swelling of tissue.
    c. Blood disorders.
    d. None of the above.

13. Blood transfusion incompatibility reactions are
    a. Potentially life threatening.
    b. Always fatal.
    c. A common problem.
    d. None of the above.

14. Lymphedema causes swelling of
    a. The heart.
    b. An extremity.
    c. Heart valves.
    d. None of the above.

15. Cardiac arrhythmias are the result of
    a. Smoking.
    b. Fat deposits.
    c. Interference with the conduction system of the heart.
    d. None of the above.

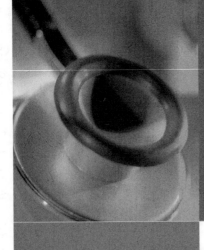

CHAPTER 11

Diseases and Conditions of the Urinary System

WORD DEFINITIONS

Define the following basic medical terms:

1. ARF _____

2. Anorexia _____

3. BUN _____

4. Calculi _____

5. Casts _____

6. Extracellular _____

7. Flank _____

8. Intrarenal _____

9. IVP _____

10. Lethargic _____

11. Nephrolithotomy _____

12. Neuropathies _____

13. Oliguria _____

14. Pitting edema _____

15. Proteinuria _____

16. Renin _____

17. Spontaneously _____

18. Urgency _____

GLOSSARY TERMS

Define the following chapter glossary terms:

1. Azotemia _____

2. BUN _____

3. Calculi _____

4. Clean-catch urine specimen _____

5. Dialysis _____

6. Erythrocyte sedimentation rate (ESR) _____

7. Fibrotic _____

8. Glomerulosclerosis _____

9. Glomeruli _____

10. Hematuria _____

11. Hypoalbuminemia _____

12. Idiopathic _____

13. Intravenous pyelograms _____

14. Intravenous urogram _____

15. Malaise _____

16. Metabolic acidosis _____

17. Nephrons _____

18. Pyelonephritis _____

19. Renal calculi _____

20. Uremia _____

SHORT ANSWER

Answer the following questions:

1. Can chronic glomerulonephritis lead to renal failure?

   _____

2. What diagnostic test is often ordered to evaluate the function of the urinary system?

   _____

3. What usually precedes acute glomerulonephritis?

   _____

4. Name the procedure used to examine the urinary tract.

   _____

5. Regardless of the size of the stone, are symptoms of renal calculi the same?

   _____

6. What is the most common type of kidney disease?

   _____

7. List causes of neurogenic bladder.

   _____

8. Describe hematuria.

   _____

9. List the functions of the urinary system.

   _____

10. Pressure from urine that cannot flow past an obstruction in the urinary tract causes what condition affecting the kidney?

    _____

11. List types of nephrotoxic agents that commonly cause renal damage.

    _____

    _____

12. Name the treatment of choice for renal cell carcinoma.

    _____

13. Define nephrotic syndrome.

    _____

14. Glomerulosclerosis results from what disease?

_____

15. List usual causes of cystitis and urethritis.

_____

_____

16. In relation to the urinary system, list the occasions when catheterization may be indicated.

_____

_____

17. Define pyuria.

_____

18. List the symptoms of acute glomerulonephritis.

_____

19. List factors that may lead to stress incontinence (enuresis).

_____

_____

20. Identify the cause of bladder cancer.

_____

21. Describe the sequence of events when a patient has acute renal failure.

_____

_____

22. After what length of time will a kidney fail to function if an obstruction is not resolved when the patient has hydronephrosis?

_____

23. Explain the usual treatment of renal calculi.

_____

24. Identify the cause of polycystic kidney disease.

_____

25. Describe the appearance of a polycystic kidney.

_____

_____

FILL IN THE BLANKS

Fill in the blanks with the correct terms. A word list has been provided. Words used twice are indicated with a (2).

1. With renal cell carcinoma, the malignancy can begin in the

   _____ or be secondary to carcinoma elsewhere in

   the body.

2. The urinary system is responsible for _____,

   _____, and _____ _____.

3. The functional unit of the kidney is the _____.

4. The three functional processes of the kidney in the manufacture

   of urine are _____, _____, and

   _____.

5. Urine is stored in the _____.

6. Function of the urinary system is evaluated by _____ and

   _____ _____.

7. Four symptoms of urinary disease are _____,

   _____ _____, _____

   _____ _____ and _____.

8. _____ _____ is an inflammation and

   swelling of the glomeruli.

9. The major structures of the urinary system consist of

   _____ _____, two _____,

   the _____ _____, and the

   _____.

10. Nephrotic syndrome encompasses a group of symptoms referred to as

    _____ _____ kidney.

11. Initial symptoms of acute renal failure include _____,

    _____ _____, _____

    _____, and other alterations in the level of consciousness.

12. The treatment of choice for pyelonephritis consists of intravenous or

    oral _____, usually _____ or

    _____, given for a full 7 to _____ days.

13. Kidney stones form when there is an excessive amount of

    _____ or _____ _____

    in the blood.

14. Diabetic patients vary in their susceptibility to renal

    _____, so the treatment plan for diabetic

    glomerulosclerosis is _____ for each person.

15. The treatment for neurogenic bladder is directed toward prevention

    of _____ and attempts to restore some

    _____ in function.

WORD LIST

10, acute glomerulonephritis, antibiotics, bladder, blood tests, bloody urine, calcium, cephalosporin, decreased urinary output, drowsiness, excreting urine, failure, filtration, gastrointestinal disturbances, headache, hypertension, individualized, kidneys (2), nausea, nephron, normalcy, oliguria, penicillin, producing, protein losing, reabsorption, secretion, storing, ureters, urethra, uric acid, urinalysis, urinary bladder, urinary tract infections (UTIs)

ANATOMIC STRUCTURES

Identify the structures in the following anatomic diagrams. For number 4, identify the three phases of urine formation.

1. The urinary system

(1) _____

(2) _____

(3) _____

(4) _____

(5) _____

(6) _____

(7) _____

(8) _____

(9) _____

(10) _____

(11) _____

(12) _____

(13) _____

(14) _____

(15) _____

(16) _____

(17) _____

2. Internal structure of the kidney

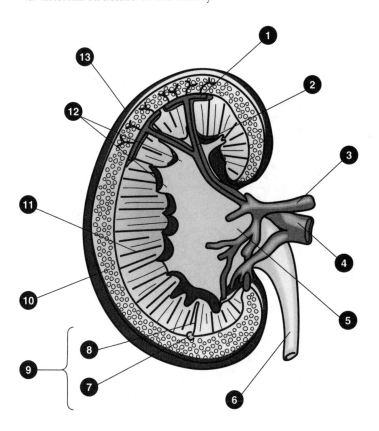

(1) _____   (8) _____

(2) _____   (9) _____

(3) _____   (10) _____

(4) _____   (11) _____

(5) _____   (12) _____

(6) _____   (13) _____

(7) _____

3. The nephron

(1) _____   (9) _____

(2) _____   (10) _____

(3) _____   (11) _____

(4) _____   (12) _____

(5) _____   (13) _____

(6) _____   (14) _____

(7) _____   (15) _____

(8) _____

4. Formation of urine

CELLS AND PROTEIN REMAIN IN BLOOD

Efferent arteriole

Glomerular capillaries

Proximal convoluted tubule

GLUCOSE
AA
Na⁺
WATER

Distal convoluted tubule

DRUGS

H⁺
K⁺

B⁻

1.

WATER

2.

Na⁺

WATER
(ADH effect)

Juxtaglomerular cells

(Aldosterone effect)

3.

Afferent arteriole

Peritubular capillaries

Na⁺
Cl⁻

Vein

Filtrate

Collecting duct

Na⁺
Cl⁻

WATER
(by osmosis)

Urine

KEY
AA   Amino acids
B⁻   Bicarbonate ions
Cl⁻ Chloride ions
H⁺   Hydrogen ions
K⁺   Potassium ions
Na⁺ Sodium ions

PATIENT SCREENING

For each scenario below, explain how and why you would schedule an appointment or suggest a referral based on the patient's reported symptoms. First, review the "Guidelines for Patient-Screening Exercises" found on page iii in the "Introduction."

1. A mother calls in reporting her daughter has experienced a sudden onset of grossly bloody urine. The urine is dark and is described as being coffee-colored. The child had a streptococcal infection 1 to 2 weeks ago. The child also is complaining of a headache, has a loss of appetite, and a low-grade fever. Flank or back pain is an additional complaint of the child. How do you handle this call?

_____

_____

_____

_____

2. A patient reports she has experienced rapid onset of fever, chills, nausea and vomiting, and flank (lumbar) pain. She had a UTI with urinary frequency and urgency last week. The patient reports a foul odor to the urine with possible blood and pus. There is tenderness in the suprapubic region. How do you handle this call?

_____

_____

_____

_____

3. A patient calls in advising he has experienced sudden severe pain in the flank area and urinary urgency. He also is complaining of nausea and vomiting, blood in the urine, fever, chills, and abdominal distention. How do you respond to this phone call?

_____

_____

_____

_____

4. A female patient calls the office complaining of urinary urgency, frequency, and even incontinence. Additionally, she says she has pain in the pelvic region and low back, spasm of the bladder, fever and chills, and a burning sensation with urination. Her urine is dark yellow. How do you respond to this phone call?

_____

_____

_____

_____

5. A female patient advises she is experiencing leakage of urine on coughing, sneezing, laughing, lifting, or running, without prior urgency. The patient is unable to control the leakage during physical exertion. How do you handle this call?

_____

_____

_____

_____

PATIENT TEACHING

For each scenario below, outline the appropriate patient teaching you would perform. First, review the "Guidelines for Patient-Teaching Exercises" found on page iv in the "Introduction."

1. ACUTE GLOMERULONEPHRITIS
   A patient has recently been diagnosed with acute glomerulonephritis. Antibiotics have been prescribed. The physician has printed instructions for patients with this condition. You are asked to provide the patient and family with the printed information and review it with them. How do you approach this patient-teaching opportunity?

_____

_____

_____

_____

2. PYELONEPHRITIS

A female patient has a recurring occurrence of pyelonephritis. The physician has requested you to provide and review this material with the patient. How do you approach this patient-teaching opportunity?

_____

_____

_____

_____

3. RENAL CALCULI

A patient complains of sudden onset of severe flank pain accompanied by pelvic pressure. Radiographs indicate the presence of renal calculi. The physician requests you to provide the patient with printed information concerning renal calculi therapy. How do you approach this patient-teaching opportunity?

_____

_____

_____

_____

4. DIABETIC NEPHROPATHY

A patient has recently been diagnosed with diabetic neuropathy. He is somewhat confused about this complication of his diabetes. The physician has written information for this type of disorder. You are instructed to provide him with the printed information and to review its contents with him. How do you approach this patient-teaching opportunity?

_____

_____

_____

_____

5. STRESS INCONTINENCE

A female patient has been experiencing stress incontinence. The physician has printed instructions to help patients deal with this condition. The physician requests that you provide the instructions to the patient and that you review them with her. How do you approach this patient-teaching opportunity?

_____

_____

_____

_____

PHARMACOLOGY QUESTIONS

Circle the letter of the choice that best completes the statement or answers the question.

1. Which of the following medications may cause nephrotoxicity?
   a. Cyclosporin (Neoral)
   b. Amphotericin B
   c. Acetaminophen (Tylenol)
   d. All of the above

2. Treatment of UTI's may include all of the following therapies except
   a. Sulfamethoxazole/trimethoprim (Bactrim).
   b. Amoxicillin (Amoxil).
   c. Reduced fluid intake.
   d. Phenazopyridine (Pyridium).

3. Urinary incontinence due to muscle spasms of the bladder may be treated with _____.
   a. Cyclobenzaprine (Flexeril)
   b. Oxybutynin (Ditropan)
   c. Tolterodine (Detrol)
   d. Both b & c

ESSAY QUESTION

Write a response to the following question or statement. Use a separate sheet of paper if more space is needed.

Compare hemodialysis and peritoneal dialysis.

_____

_____

_____

_____

_____

_____

_____

_____

_____

_____

_____

_____

_____

_____

_____

_____

CERTIFICATION EXAMINATION REVIEW

Circle the letter of the choice that best completes the statement or answers the question.

1. Obstructive diseases of the kidney may be caused by
   a. Metabolic disorders.
   b. Congenital or structural defects.
   c. Immunologic disorders.
   d. None of the above.

2. The most common type of renal disease is
   a. Acute renal failure.
   b. Nephrosis.
   c. Pyelonephritis.
   d. Hydronephrosis.

3. Symptoms of cystitis include
   a. Urinary urgency, frequency, and incontinence.
   b. Pelvic pain.
   c. Burning with urination.
   d. All of the above.

4. Group A beta hemolytic streptococcus may precede
   a. Hydronephrosis.
   b. Acute renal failure.
   c. Acute glomerulonephritis.
   d. None of the above.

5. Lithotripsy, relief of pain, surgical intervention, increased fluid intake, and diuretics are all ways of treating
   a. Hydronephrosis.
   b. Renal calculi.
   c. Glomerulonephritis.
   d. All of the above.

6. An ascending bacterial invasion of the urinary tract can cause
   a. Renal calculi.
   b. Hydronephrosis.
   c. Cystitis and urethritis.
   d. All of the above.

7. Chronic glomerulonephritis is
   a. Slowly progressive and infectious.
   b. Slowly progressive and noninfectious.
   c. Not progressive.
   d. None of the above.

8. Enuresis is caused from a weakening of
   a. The pelvic floor muscles.
   b. The urethral structure.
   c. Both a and b.
   d. None of the above.

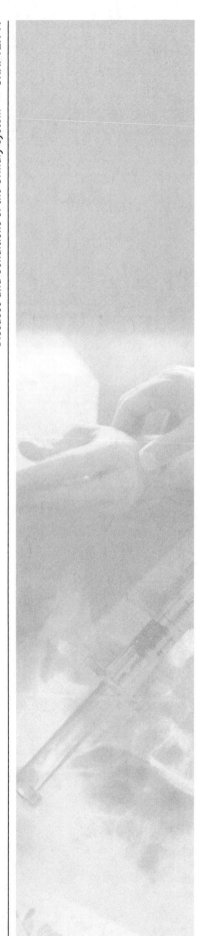

9. Solvents, heavy metals, antibiotics, pesticides, and mushrooms are known to
   a. Cause renal damage.
   b. Cause cystitis.
   c. Cause pyelonephritis.
   d. None of the above.

10. Smoking, obesity, and prolonged exposure to chemicals, such as asbestos and cadmium, may cause
    a. Polycystic kidney disease.
    b. Renal cell carcinoma.
    c. Glomerulonephritis.
    d. None of the above.

11. Pus in the urine is called
    a. Azotemia.
    b. Pyuria.
    c. Cystitis.
    d. None of the above.

12. Hematuria is
    a. Bacteria in the urine.
    b. Blood in the urine.
    c. Fat in the urine.
    d. None of the above.

13. Azotemia is
    a. A drug that promotes urine output.
    b. Excess urea in the blood.
    c. Excess urea in the urine.
    d. None of the above.

14. A clinical emergency that involves the renal system is
    a. Cystitis.
    b. Hematuria.
    c. Acute renal failure.
    d. Pyuria.

CHAPTER 12

Diseases and Conditions of the Reproductive System

WORD DEFINITIONS

Define the following basic medical terms:

1. Amenorrhea _____

2. Anomaly _____

3. Axillary _____

4. Cervicitis _____

5. Cystitis _____

6. Cystoscopy _____

7. Degenerative _____

8. Endometrial _____

9. Lymphectomy _____

10. Melena _____

11. Nocturia _____

12. Noninvasive _____

13. Proctoscopy _____

14. Prostatitis _____

15. Septicemia _____

16. Urethritis _____

GLOSSARY TERMS

Define the following chapter glossary terms:

1. Abruptio placentae _____

2. Amniotic fluid _____

3. Asymptomatic _____

4. Colporrhaphy _____

5. Endometrium _____

6. Laparoscopy _____

7. Neoplasm _____

8. Nulliparous _____

9. Pathologist _____

10. Peau d'orange _____

11. Pelvic
    inflammatory disease _____

12. Peritonitis _____

13. Prostate-
    specific antigen _____

14. Serologic _____

15. Zygote _____

SHORT ANSWER

Answer the following questions:

1. Name the male reproductive organs that produce sperm.

    _____

2. Identify the drug of choice to treat syphilis.

    _____

3. List the signs and symptoms of preeclampsia in pregnancy.

    _____

    _____

4. Identify the first sign of testicular cancer.

    _____

5. What is dysmenorrhea?

_____

6. Name the term for pain that occurs at ovulation.

_____

7. Name the sexually transmitted disease that is referred to as the "silent STD."

_____

8. Identify the treatment for condylomata.

_____

9. What happens during placenta previa?

_____

10. Identify the second leading cause of cancer deaths among women.

_____

11. What is the best prevention of epididymitis?

_____

12. Identify the treatment for testicular torsion.

_____

13. List complications of benign prostatic hypertrophy.

_____

14. Testicular cancer is most common in men of what age?

_____

15. Cite causes of secondary dysmenorrhea.

_____

16. What is a leiomyoma?

_____

17. What is included in the diagnostic evaluation for prostatic cancer?

_____

_____

18. Is dyspareunia more common in men or women?

_____

19. Identify the main goals of treatment for genital herpes.

_____

20. By what route is genital herpes transmitted?

_____

21. Are physical problems always the cause of impotence?

_____

22. With regular unprotected intercourse for 1 year, what percentage of couples is able to conceive?

_____

23. What is the age range in which most women are diagnosed with ovarian cancer?

_____

24. Identify the time during pregnancy that most women experience morning sickness.

_____

25. With ectopic pregnancy, where does the fertilized ovum usually implant?

_____

26. List the characteristics of eclampsia.

_____

27. What is the difference between a complete and incomplete hydatidiform mole?

_____

28. Is cystic disease of the breast benign or cancerous?

_____

FILL IN THE BLANKS

Fill in the blanks with the correct terms. A word list has been provided.

1. Sperm is transported from the testes through the series of ducts

    beginning with the epididymis, the _____, and the

    _____ ducts.

2. The _____ are accessory organs of _____

    and are two milk-producing glands.

3. Sexually transmitted disease (STD) rates in the _____ are

    among the highest in the world and are growing.

4. Trichomoniasis is a _____ infection of the

    _____ genitourinary tract.

5. Genital warts are usually painless, but they may _____ or _____.

6. The most common diseases of the male reproductive system are those affecting the _____ gland.

7. _____ or _____ infection or _____ causes inflammation of the testes.

8. In endometriosis _____ tissue grows outside of the _____ cavity.

9. Leiomyomas are the most common _____ of the female reproductive system.

10. Toxic shock syndrome is an _____, _____ infection with toxin producing _____ of *Staphylococcus aureus*.

11. Many _____ experience the onset of menopause between the ages of _____ and _____.

12. Prolapse of the uterus is a _____ displacement of the _____ from its normal location in the pelvis.

13. A _____ is a downward displacement of the urinary bladder into the _____ wall of the vagina.

14. Exercises to strengthen the pelvic floor muscles are called _____ exercises.

15. Mastitis is frequently caused by a _____ or _____ infection.

WORD LIST

45, 55, acute, anterior, bacterial, breast, burn, cystocele, downward, ductus deferens, ejaculatory, endometrial, injury, itch, Kegel, lower, prostate, protozoal, reproduction, staphylococcal, strains, streptococcal, systemic, tumors, United States, uterine, uterus, viral, women

ANATOMIC STRUCTURES

Identify the structures in the following anatomic diagrams.

1. Normal male reproductive system

(1) _____   (7) _____

(2) _____   (8) _____

(3) _____   (9) _____

(4) _____   (10) _____

(5) _____   (11) _____

(6) _____   (12) _____

2. Normal female reproductive system

(1) _____

(2) _____

(3) _____

(4) _____

(5) _____

(6) _____

(7) _____

(8) _____

(9) _____

(10) _____

(11) _____

(12) _____

3. Normal female breast

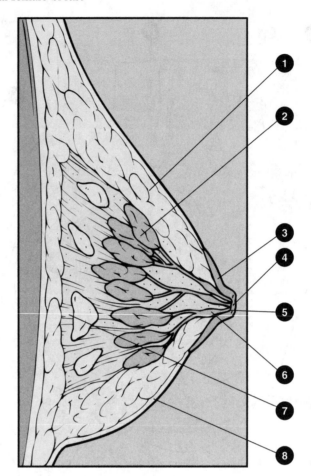

(1) _____

(2) _____

(3) _____

(4) _____

(5) _____

(6) _____

(7) _____

(8) _____

PATIENT SCREENING

For each scenario below, explain how and why you would schedule an appointment or suggest a referral based on the patient's reported symptoms. First, review the "Guidelines for Patient-Screening Exercises" found on page iii in the "Introduction."

1. A female patient calls in requesting an appointment saying she is experiencing painful urination and severe itching in the perineal region. How do you respond to her call?

_____

_____

_____

2. A 60-year-old male patient calls the office advising he is experiencing urinary frequency including nocturia. How do you handle this call?

_____

_____

_____

3. A female patient calls advising she is experiencing fever, chills, a foul-smelling vaginal discharge, backache, and a painful, tender abdomen. How do you handle this call?

_____

_____

_____

4. A female patient's husband calls the office saying his wife is 2 months pregnant and has developed vaginal bleeding and pelvic pain from cramping. How do you handle this call?

_____

_____

_____

5. A female patient calls in requesting an appointment stating she has been experiencing an uncomfortable feeling in her breasts. She found a lump this morning in her right breast. How do you handle this call?

_____

_____

_____

Diseases and Conditions of the Reproductive System ■ **CHAPTER 12**

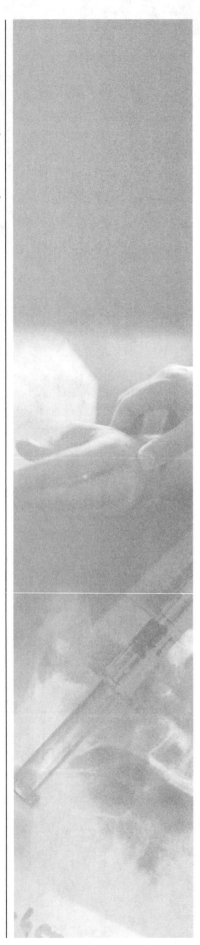

PATIENT TEACHING

For each scenario below, outline the appropriate patient teaching you would perform. First, review the "Guidelines for Patient-Teaching Exercises" found on page iv in the "Introduction."

1. SYPHILIS
   A patient has been diagnosed with syphilis. The practice has printed instructions for patients diagnosed with this condition. The physician has instructed you to provide the patient with the printed information and to review it with her. How do you approach this patient-teaching opportunity?

   _____

   _____

   _____

   _____

   _____

   _____

2. ORCHITIS
   A young male patient has just been diagnosed with orchitis. The physician requests you provide the patient with the printed information concerning this condition. How do you approach this patient-teaching opportunity?

   _____

   _____

   _____

   _____

   _____

3. PREMENSTRUAL SYNDROME (PMS)
   A female patient complains of typical premenstrual syndrome symptoms. The office has printed information for patient teaching about this condition. The physician requests you to provide the information sheets to the patient and review them with her. How do you approach this patient-teaching opportunity?

   _____

   _____

   _____

   _____

   _____

4. **ENDOMETRIOSIS**

   A young female patient has been complaining of intolerable menstrual cramps and other pelvic pain. The diagnosis of endometriosis has been made. The physician has written instructions for this condition. You are instructed to provide the patient with the printed material and review it with her. How do you approach this patient-teaching opportunity?

   _____

   _____

   _____

   _____

   _____

5. **PREECLAMPSIA (TOXEMIA)**

   A pregnant patient has been experiencing elevated blood pressure and sudden weight gain. She has been diagnosed with preeclampsia. The physician has printed instructions for this condition. You are instructed to provide this information to the patient and her family. How do you approach this patient-teaching opportunity?

   _____

   _____

   _____

   _____

   _____

PHARMACOLOGY QUESTIONS

Circle the letter of the choice that best completes the statement or answers the question.

1. Treatment of gonorrhea has become more complex due to antibiotic resistance to which antibiotic?
   a. Penicillin
   b. Amoxicillin
   c. Tetracycline
   d. All of the above

2. Genital herpes is not curable, but drug therapy may reduce the frequency and duration of outbreaks. Which medication(s) is(are) frequently used to treat this disease?
   a. Acyclovir (Zovirax)
   b. Famciclovir (Famvir)
   c. Valacyclovir (Valtrex)
   d. All of the above

3. Which of the following statements are associated with the use of sildenafil (Viagra)?
   a. Men who have had a heart attack should not take Viagra.
   b. Viagra may cause temporary vision changes (blurred vision or color changes).
   c. Both of the above
   d. Neither of the above

4. Benign prostatic hyperplasia (BPH) is a common condition of men 50 years and older. Which of the following medications should be avoided with this condition?
   a. Pseudoephedrine (Sudafed)
   b. Doxazosin (Cardura)
   c. Finasteride (Proscar)
   d. Tamsulosin (Flomax)

5. Which of the following may be useful in the treatment of menopause?
   a. Conjugated hormone (Premarin)
   b. Alendronate (Fosamax)
   c. Weight-bearing exercise
   d. All of the above

6. Drug catagories for reproductive hormone replacement include
   a. Androgens.
   b. Estrogens.
   c. Progestins.
   d. All of the above.

ESSAY QUESTION

Write a response to the following question or statement. Use a separate sheet of paper if more space is needed.

Discuss the cause, symptoms and signs, and treatment of premature labor.

_____

_____

_____

_____

_____

_____

_____

_____

_____

_____

_____

_____

_____

CERTIFICATION EXAMINATION REVIEW

Circle the letter of the choice that best completes the statement or answers the question.

1. Genital warts and many different types of cancer develop from
    a. Syphilis.
    b. Human papillomavirus (HPV).
    c. Chlamydia.
    d. None of the above.

2. Pelvic inflammatory disease, septicemia, and septic arthritis are complications that may develop from untreated
    a. Syphilis.
    b. HPV.
    c. Gonorrhea.
    d. None of the above.

3. When functioning endometrial tissue is present outside the uterine cavity, the condition is called _____.
    a. Septicemia
    b. Gonorrhea
    c. Uterine cancer
    d. None of the above

4. Dyspareunia is more common in
    a. Men.
    b. Women.
    c. Teenagers.
    d. Toddlers.

5. Impotence may be caused from
    a. Use of recreational drugs.
    b. Use of hypertensive medications.
    c. Drinking alcohol.
    d. All of the above.

6. Protrusion of the rectum into the bladder is a
    a. Cystocele.
    b. Rectal fissure.
    c. Rectocele.
    d. None of the above.

7. Pain that occurs at ovulation is called
    a. Premenstrual syndrome.
    b. Mittelschmerz
    c. Both a and b.
    d. None of the above.

8. A Pap smear may be a valuable tool in diagnosing
    a. Cervical cancer.
    b. Breast cancer.
    c. Testicular cancer.
    d. All of the above.

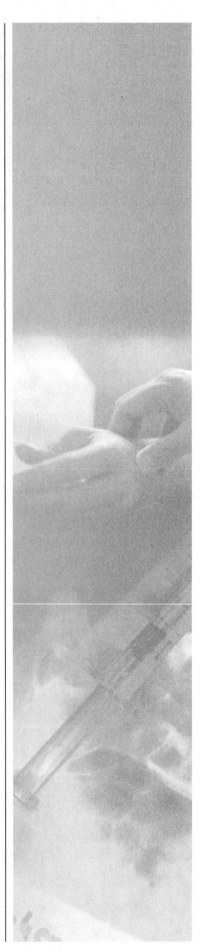

9. Herpes simplex virus
   a. Is not curable.
   b. Is easily treated.
   c. Is only detected by a Pap smear.
   d. None of the above.

10. A digital rectal examination, blood test for prostate-specific antigen (PSA), and a biopsy to confirm are all evaluations for
   a. Prostate cancer.
   b. Testicular cancer.
   c. Bladder cancer.
   d. None of the above.

11. Signs of hyperemesis gravidarum may include
   a. Dehydration.
   b. Abnormal urinalysis.
   c. Abnormal blood chemistries.
   d. All of the above.

12. Premenstrual dysphoric disorder (PMDD) refers to
   a. Toxemia.
   b. Chlamydia.
   c. Morning sickness.
   d. Severe premenstrual syndrome (PMS)

13. Human papillomavirus (HPV) vaccine is
   a. A major advance in the prevention of cervical cancer.
   b. Recommended for girls and women 9 to 26 years of age.
   c. Given as three doses at 0, 2, and 6 months.
   d. All of the above.

CHAPTER 13

Neurologic Diseases and Conditions

WORD DEFINITIONS

Define the following basic medical terms:

1. Bradycardia   _____

2. Cephalgia   _____

3. Craniotomy   _____

4. Dilated   _____

5. Dysarthric   _____

6. Empyema   _____

7. Flaccid   _____

8. Hemicranial   _____

9. Hemiparesis   _____

10. Hypotension   _____

11. Intervertebral   _____

12. Intracranial   _____

13. Laminectomy   _____

14. Photophobia   _____

15. Sequela   _____

16. Syncope   _____

GLOSSARY TERMS

Define the following chapter glossary terms:

1. Autosomal _____

2. Cauterize _____

3. Demyelination _____

4. Diplopia _____

5. Encephalitis _____

6. Ergot _____

7. Fibrin _____

8. Foramen _____

9. Hemiparesis _____

10. Intractable _____

11. Lumbar puncture _____

12. Neurotransmitter _____

13. Nuchal rigidity _____

14. Paresis _____

15. Plasmapheresis _____

SHORT ANSWER

Answer the following questions:

1. Identify the difference between efferent and afferent nerves.

   _____

   _____

2. Identify the cause of cerebrovascular accidents.

   _____

   _____

3. Cite another name for a transient ischemic attack (TIA).

   _____

4. Does a TIA usually cause unconsciousness?

   _____

5. Which is more serious, a concussion or a cerebral contusion?

_____

6. Identify the common complication of a depressed skull fracture.

_____

_____

7. Identify the most frequent cause of a depressed skull.

_____

_____

8. What is the goal of treatment for spinal cord injuries?

_____

_____

9. List the symptoms of degenerative disk disease.

_____

_____

_____

10. Name the function of an intervertebral disk.

_____

11. Is sciatic nerve injury considered a pathologic condition?

_____

12. If a person is having seizures, does it always mean they have epilepsy?

_____

13. Identify the type of medications that are used to treat epilepsy.

_____

14. Encephalitis is usually the result of a bite from what insect?

_____

15. List possible treatments for a brain abscess.

_____

16. Explain why a lumbar puncture is contraindicated if the patient has a brain abscess.

_____

17. Identify the symptoms of Guillain-Barré syndrome.

_____

_____

18. Identify the vaccines that have helped eliminate cases of poliomyelitis.

_____

19. Cite the statistics for overall 5-year survival of all types of brain tumors.

_____

20. Identify the area of the skull involved with a basilar skull fracture.

_____

21. What physical manifestations alert the physician to order images of the cranial vault to investigate for a basilar skull fracture?

_____

22. Name the possible routes through which the poliomyelitis virus may enter the body.

_____

23. How are primary brain tumors classified?

_____

24. Identify the race having the highest incidence of brain tumors.

_____

25. How are the cranial nerves assessed during a neurologic examination?

_____

Fill in the Blanks

Fill in the blanks with the correct terms. A word list has been provided. Words used twice are indicated with a (2).

1. Electrical impulses are carried throughout the body by

_____.

2. The two divisions of the nervous system are the _____

nervous system and the _____ nervous system.

3. The central nervous system (CNS) includes the _____

and _____ _____.

4. Five pairs of the _____ cranial nerves originate in the _____ _____, an extension of the spinal cord.

5. The _____ is divided into 31 segments.

6. A cerebral concussion is a _____ of the cerebral tissue that is caused by _____ back and forth movement of the head as in an acceleration-deceleration insult.

7. A contusion of the brain is caused by a _____ to the _____ or an _____ against a hard surface, as in an automobile accident.

8. When a portion of the skull is broken and pushed in on the brain, causing injury, it is said to be a _____ skull fracture.

9. Quadriplegia results in paralysis of the _____ _____ and usually the trunk.

10. Intervertebral disks are soft pads of _____ located between each vertebrae that make up the _____.

11. Headaches may be acute or chronic and located in the _____ _____, _____, or _____ _____ regions of the head.

12. Before the onset of a headache, many persons who experience _____ headaches have visual auras.

13. Partial seizures do not involve the _____ _____ brain but arise from a _____ _____ area in the brain.

14. Anticonvulsant medications are the treatment of choice for _____ _____ _____ _____.

15. Patients with amyotrophic lateral sclerosis (ALS) have difficulty with speech, _____, _____, and _____, and eventually will require a ventilator.

WORD LIST

12, blow, brain, breathing, bruising, cartilage, central, chewing, depressed, entire, epilepsy, frontal, head, impact, localized, lower extremities, medulla oblongata, migraine, neurons, occipital, peripheral, spinal cord (2), spine, swallowing, temporal, violent

ANATOMIC STRUCTURES

Identify the structures in the following anatomic diagrams. For number 8, identify the type of paralysis each illustration represents.

1. The normal brain

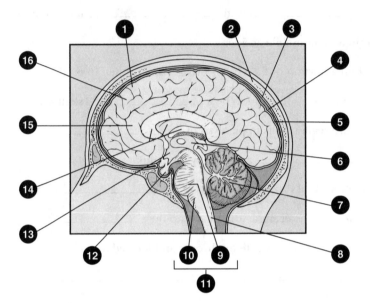

(1) _____   (9) _____

(2) _____   (10) _____

(3) _____   (11) _____

(4) _____   (12) _____

(5) _____   (13) _____

(6) _____   (14) _____

(7) _____   (15) _____

(8) _____   (16) _____

2. The spinal cord

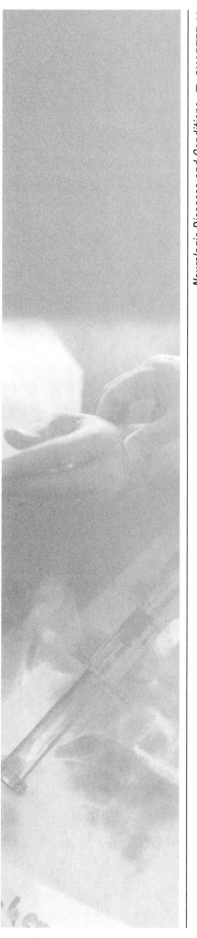

(1) _____

(2) _____

(3) _____

(4) _____

(5) _____

3. The neuron

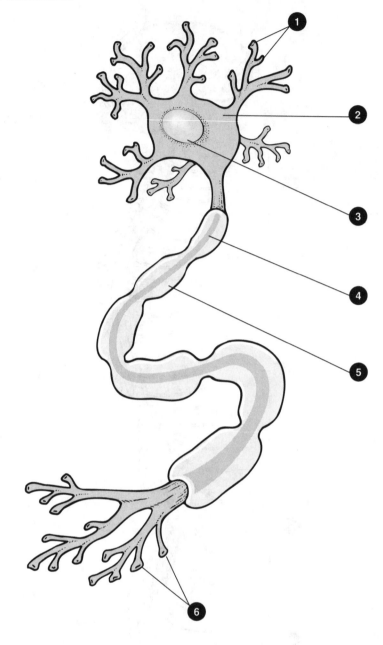

(1) _____

(2) _____

(3) _____

(4) _____

(5) _____

(6) _____

4. Functional areas of the brain

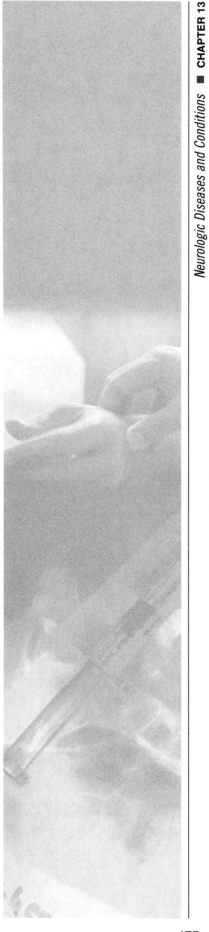

(1) _____   (15) _____

(2) _____   (16) _____

(3) _____   (17) _____

(4) _____   (18) _____

(5) _____   (19) _____

(6) _____   (20) _____

(7) _____   (21) _____

(8) _____   (22) _____

(9) _____   (23) _____

(10) _____   (24) _____

(11) _____   (25) _____

(12) _____   (26) _____

(13) _____   (27) _____

(14) _____   (28) _____

5. The peripheral nervous system

MAJOR NERVES OF SHOULDER

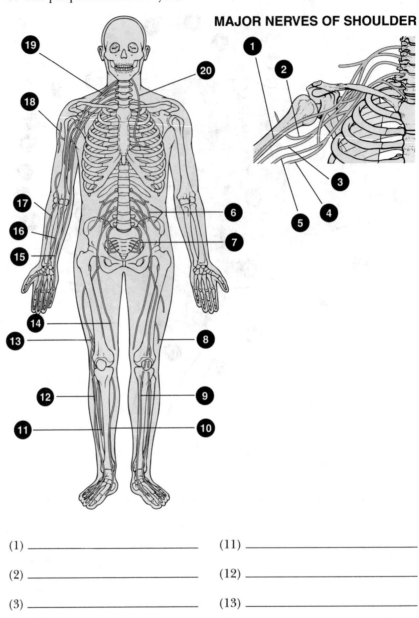

(1) _____   (11) _____

(2) _____   (12) _____

(3) _____   (13) _____

(4) _____   (14) _____

(5) _____   (15) _____

(6) _____   (16) _____

(7) _____   (17) _____

(8) _____   (18) _____

(9) _____   (19) _____

(10) _____   (20) _____

6. The cranial nerves

(1) _____   (13) _____

(2) _____   (14) _____

(3) _____   (15) _____

(4) _____   (16) _____

(5) _____   (17) _____

(6) _____   (18) _____

(7) _____   (19) _____

(8) _____   (20) _____

(9) _____   (21) _____

(10) _____   (22) _____

(11) _____   (23) _____

(12) _____

7. Major arteries of the head and neck

(1) _____

(2) _____

(3) _____

(4) _____

(5) _____

(6) _____

(7) _____

8. Types of paralysis

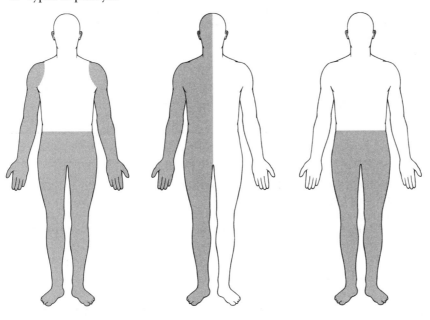

_____   _____   _____

PATIENT SCREENING

For each scenario below, explain how and why you would schedule an appointment or suggest a referral based on the patient's reported symptoms. First, review the "Guidelines for Patient-Screening Exercises" found on page iii in the "Introduction."

1. A patient's wife calls in reporting her husband is experiencing weakness and numbness down one side of the body, dizziness, and confusion. He is conscious. How do you respond to this call?

   _____

   _____

   _____

   _____

2. The mother of a 12-year-old boy calls the office and tells you her son fell down the stairs and experienced an immediate loss of consciousness. This episode lasted for approximately 5 minutes. He has regained consciousness and is experiencing a headache, nausea, vomiting, blurred vision, and photophobia (sensitivity to light). He also is irritable. How do you handle this call?

   _____

   _____

   _____

   _____

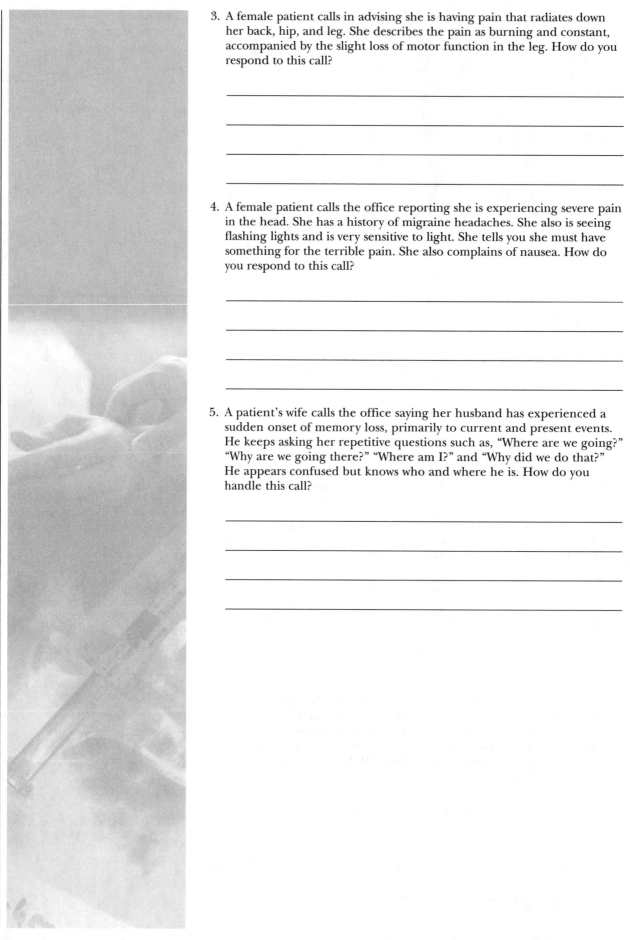

3. A female patient calls in advising she is having pain that radiates down her back, hip, and leg. She describes the pain as burning and constant, accompanied by the slight loss of motor function in the leg. How do you respond to this call?

_____

_____

_____

_____

4. A female patient calls the office reporting she is experiencing severe pain in the head. She has a history of migraine headaches. She also is seeing flashing lights and is very sensitive to light. She tells you she must have something for the terrible pain. She also complains of nausea. How do you respond to this call?

_____

_____

_____

_____

5. A patient's wife calls the office saying her husband has experienced a sudden onset of memory loss, primarily to current and present events. He keeps asking her repetitive questions such as, "Where are we going?" "Why are we going there?" "Where am I?" and "Why did we do that?" He appears confused but knows who and where he is. How do you handle this call?

_____

_____

_____

_____

PATIENT TEACHING

For each scenario below, outline the appropriate patient teaching you would perform. First, review the "Guidelines for Patient-Teaching Exercises" found on page iv in the "Introduction."

1. CEREBROVASCULAR ACCIDENT (CVA) AND TRANSIENT ISCHEMIC ATTACK (TIA)

    These patients usually have been seen in an emergency facility and have come to the office for follow-up care. The physician has printed information regarding both conditions and comparison of the conditions. You are requested to provide this information to a patient and family who have experienced CVA or TIA. How do you approach this patient-teaching opportunity?

    _____

    _____

    _____

    _____

    _____

    _____

2. HEAD INJURY

    A patient has experienced a traumatic insult to the head. He has been released from the emergency facility and is in the office for follow-up care. The physician has printed material about closed head injuries. You are instructed by the physician to provide this information to the patient and family members. How do you proceed with this patient-teaching opportunity?

    _____

    _____

    _____

    _____

    _____

    _____

3. **RUPTURED DISK**

A patient has been experiencing severe lower back pain. A diagnosis of ruptured lumbar disk has been made. You are instructed by the physician to provide printed information to the patient. How do you handle this patient-teaching opportunity?

_____

_____

_____

_____

_____

_____

4. **MIGRAINE HEADACHE**

A patient has been diagnosed with a migraine headache. The physician has printed instructions for therapy for this condition. You have been instructed to review these instructions with the patient and give her a copy of the information. How do you handle this patient-teaching opportunity?

_____

_____

_____

_____

_____

_____

5. **PARKINSON'S DISEASE**

A patient was recently diagnosed with Parkinson's disease. The physician has written instructions and information concerning this condition. The physician requests you provide and review the printed information with the patient and family. How do you handle this patient-teaching opportunity?

_____

_____

_____

_____

_____

_____

Pharmacology Questions

Circle the letter of the choice that best completes the statement or answers the question.

1. Treatment of stroke may include which of the following medications?
   a. Aspirin
   b. Metaproterenol (Lopressor)
   c. Lisinopril (Zestril)
   d. Diazepam (Valium)

2. Migraine headaches have been treated with many different types of therapy. Which of the following is *not* a common therapy of migraine treatment?
   a. Sumatriptan (Imitrex)
   b. Propranolol (Inderal)
   c. Dipyridamole (Persantine)
   d. Ibuprofen (Motrin)

3. Which of the following is *not* considered a medication for the treatment of epilepsy?
   a. Phenobarbital
   b. Valproic acid (Depakote)
   c. Phenytoin (Dilantin)
   d. Gemfibrozil (Lopid)

4. Which of the following drug combinations is frequently used in the treatment of Parkinson's disease?
   a. Phenytoin/phenobarbital
   b. Carbidopa/levodopa
   c. Diazepam/lorazepam
   d. Atenolol/hydrochlorothiazide

Essay Questions

Write a response to the following question or statement. Use a separate sheet of paper if more space is needed.

Compare and contrast subdural and epidural hematomas.

_____

_____

_____

_____

_____

_____

_____

_____

_____

_____

Neurologic Diseases and Conditions ■ **CHAPTER 13**

_____

_____

_____

_____

_____

_____

_____

_____

_____

_____

_____

_____

_____

_____

_____

CERTIFICATION EXAMINATION REVIEW

Circle the letter of the choice that best completes the statement or answers the question.

1. Efferent nerves transmit impulses
   a. Away from the brain and spinal cord.
   b. Toward the brain and spinal cord.
   c. Both a and b.
   d. Neither a or b.

2. Afferent nerves
   a. Transmit impulses away from the brain and spinal cord.
   b. Transmit impulses toward the brain and spinal cord.
   c. Are motor nerves.
   d. Both a and c.

3. Chronic alcohol intoxication, toxicity, and infectious disease are possible causes of
   a. Neuroblastoma.
   b. Trigeminal neuralgia.
   c. Peripheral neuritis.
   d. None of the above.

4. A TIA is a _____ episode of impaired neurologic functioning due to a lack of blood flow to a portion of the brain.
   a. Permanent
   b. Chronic
   c. Temporary
   d. None of the above

5. Paraplegia is paralysis that involves loss of motor and sensory control of the trunk and
   a. One extremity.
   b. Two extremities.
   c. Four extremities.
   d. None of the above.

6. Pill rolling tremor of thumb and forefinger, muscular rigidity, masklike facial expression, and shuffling gait are all signs of
   a. Bell's palsy.
   b. Parkinson's disease.
   c. Epilepsy.
   d. None of the above.

7. The blood, penetrating trauma, and infection in adjoining structures, such as the ear or sinuses, are all routes in which infectious organisms
   a. May reach the brain and cause infection.
   b. May reach the brain and cause a stroke.
   c. May reach the brain and cause a subdural hematoma.
   d. None of the above.

8. Meningitis is an inflammation of the
   a. Brain.
   b. Spinal cord.
   c. Membranes covering the brain and spinal cord.
   d. Both a and b.

9. Poliomyelitis
   a. Is not diagnosed as frequently as it was before 1960.
   b. Is a highly contagious viral disease that affects the anterior horn cells of the gray matter in the spinal cord.
   c. Is a bacterial disease.
   d. Both a and b.

10. The prognosis for patients with tumors involving the brain is
    a. Poor.
    b. Always death.
    c. Good.
    d. Difficult to project.

11. Migraine headaches
    a. Are periodic.
    b. Are sometimes incapacitating.
    c. May be triggered by certain foods in some patients.
    d. All of the above.

12. Hemiparesis is a paralysis involving
    a. One extremity.
    b. Four extremities.
    c. Either half of the body.
    d. None of the above.

13. Huntington's chorea is a(n)
    a. Disorder caused by an infection.
    b. Inherited disorder.
    c. Characterized by dancelike movements.
    d. Both b and c.

14. Amyotrophic lateral sclerosis causes symptoms of
    a. Pill rolling and shuffling of feet.
    b. Progressive destruction of motor neurons resulting in muscle atrophy.
    c. Dancelike movements and a decline in mental function.
    d. None of the above.

Neurologic Diseases and Conditions ■ **CHAPTER 13**

185

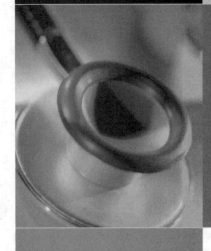

CHAPTER 14

Mental Disorders

WORD DEFINITIONS

Define the following basic medical terms:

1. Aberration   _____

2. Delusion   _____

3. Detoxification   _____

4. Febrile   _____

5. Genitourinary   _____

6. Intermittent   _____

7. Intramuscular   _____

8. Lethargy   _____

9. MRI   _____

10. Musculoskeletal   _____

11. Neurochemical   _____

12. Neurotic   _____

13. Postulated   _____

14. Precipitate   _____

15. Spontaneously   _____

GLOSSARY TERMS

Define the following chapter glossary terms:

1. Amnesia _____

2. Amyloid _____

3. Anxiolytic _____

4. Aphonia _____

5. Catatonic posturing _____

6. Continuous positive airway pressure _____

7. Hallucination _____

8. Hyperesthesia _____

9. Mutism _____

10. Paresthesia _____

11. Positron emission tomography (PET) _____

12. Prodromal _____

13. Pseudoneurologic _____

14. Ventricular shift _____

SHORT ANSWER

Answer the following questions:

1. Name the anxiety disorder that is caused from an overwhelmingly painful external event.

   _____

   _____

2. Identify the progressive degenerative disease of the brain in which there is a typical profile in the loss of mental and physical functioning. (It is the most frequent cause of deterioration of intellectual capacity or dementia.)

   _____

3. Is the specific cause of mental illness always identified?

   _____

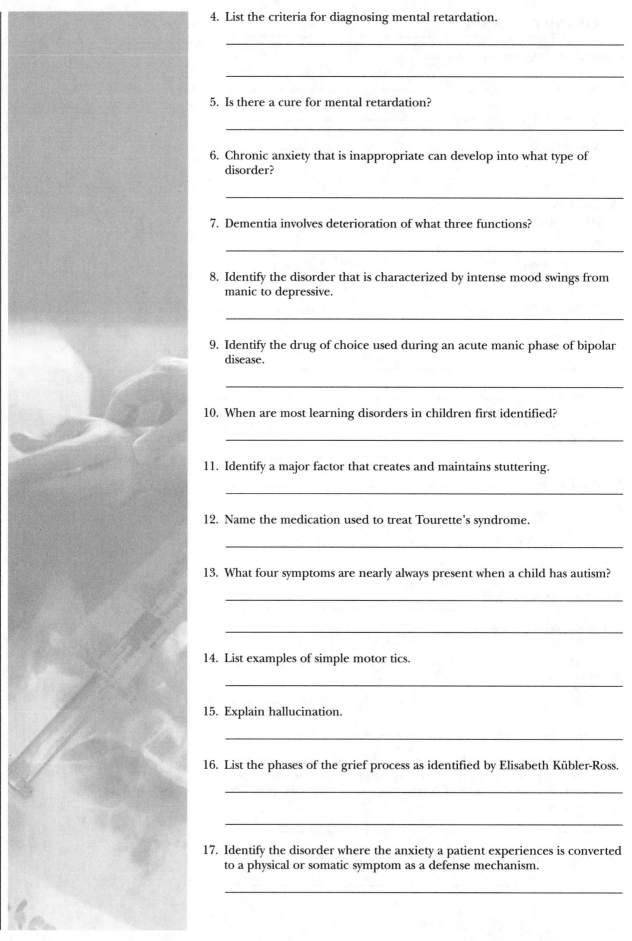

4. List the criteria for diagnosing mental retardation.

   _____

   _____

5. Is there a cure for mental retardation?

   _____

6. Chronic anxiety that is inappropriate can develop into what type of disorder?

   _____

7. Dementia involves deterioration of what three functions?

   _____

8. Identify the disorder that is characterized by intense mood swings from manic to depressive.

   _____

9. Identify the drug of choice used during an acute manic phase of bipolar disease.

   _____

10. When are most learning disorders in children first identified?

    _____

11. Identify a major factor that creates and maintains stuttering.

    _____

12. Name the medication used to treat Tourette's syndrome.

    _____

13. What four symptoms are nearly always present when a child has autism?

    _____

    _____

14. List examples of simple motor tics.

    _____

15. Explain hallucination.

    _____

16. List the phases of the grief process as identified by Elisabeth Kübler-Ross.

    _____

    _____

17. Identify the disorder where the anxiety a patient experiences is converted to a physical or somatic symptom as a defense mechanism.

    _____

18. Name the associative subtypes of pain disorders.

_____

_____

19. Identify the type of preoccupation a patient suffering from hypochondriasis experiences.

_____

20. A patient who is fully aware they are not sick or ill, but seeks medical attention anyway, would be having symptoms of which condition?

_____

21. Do somatoform disorders include a group of mental disorders where physical symptoms have an organic cause?

_____

22. Identify the test that is used to assess sleep disorders.

_____

23. To be diagnosed with insomnia, how long must sleeplessness endure?

_____

24. Identify the group of sleep disorders that include sleepwalking, night terrors, and nightmares.

_____

25. At what blood alcohol level would a person exhibit the following effects: impairment in coordination, judgment, memory, and comprehension? (Hint: In some states the person would be considered legally drunk.)

_____

26. Identify the phobia associated with a fear of blood.

_____

27. Name the phobia associated with a fear of disease.

_____

28. A person with a narcissistic personality would demonstrate what type of behavior?

_____

FILL IN THE BLANKS

Fill in the blanks with the correct terms. A word list has been provided. Words used twice are indicated with a (2).

1. Stress is considered a _____ _____ of mental disorders.

2. Mental illness has been _____ to the patient's _____ to _____ with stress imposed by _____ society.

3. Psychological pain is _____ and _____ and can _____ physical health.

4. Modern therapeutic approaches include control of symptoms with _____ _____ including antipsychotic drugs, _____, anxiolytics, CNS _____, and antimanic agents; hospitalization during _____ episodes; psychotherapy; _____ therapy and group therapy.

5. Play therapy is included in _____ for some _____.

6. Mental illnesses are categorized by _____. Each axis represents a _____ part of the diagnosis.

7. Mental retardation, or _____, is not a disease but a wide range of conditions with many causes.

8. Signs of mental retardation may be evident on well-baby _____ or during _____ checkups.

9. Mental retardation has _____, many of which are unidentifiable.

10. Learning disabilities occur when _____ learn things _____ in a manner that is _____ normal.

11. The person with learning disorders exhibits _____ in acquiring a _____ in a specific area of learning such as _____, _____, and _____.

12. Schizophrenia is _____; therefore there is no known _____.

13. Suicide intervention is an attempt by _____, mental
    health, and community services to assist the depressed individual through
    the _____ situation.

14. Personality disorders typically begin in _____.

15. Avoidance personality disorder avoids any _____ situation
    because of _____ of criticism, disapproval, or rejection.

16. Individuals with schizoid personality disorder appear to lack or show
    emotion of _____ or _____.

WORD LIST

acute, adolescence, antidepressants, axis, children (2), contributing factor,
cope, counseling, developmental disability, different, differently, difficulty,
electroconvulsive, examinations, fear, genetic, hopeless, inability, influence,
intense, linked, mathematics, medical, modern, not, numerous causes, pain,
pleasure, preschool routine, prevention, psychotropic drugs, reading, real,
skill, social, stimulants, writing

PATIENT SCREENING

For each scenario below, explain how and why you would schedule an appointment or
suggest a referral based on the patient's reported symptoms. First, review the "Guidelines
for Patient-Screening Exercises" found on page iii in the "Introduction."

1. A father calls the office saying his 6-year-old son is experiencing a speech
   pattern of frequent repetitions or prolongations of sounds or syllables.
   The fluency of his normal speech is punctuated with broken words and
   word repetitions. How do you respond to this call?

   _____

   _____

   _____

   _____

2. The daughter of an older patient calls in saying her father is
   experiencing loss of short-term memory, the inability to concentrate,
   impairment of reasoning, and subtle changes in personality. He also is
   restless, is having trouble sleeping, and is combative. How do you handle
   this call?

   _____

   _____

   _____

   _____

3. A female patient calls the office stating she is experiencing deep and persistent sadness, despair, and hopelessness. She says she is having problems sleeping and does not want to eat. This started a few days ago and is getting worse. She wants help. How do you handle this call?

_____

_____

_____

_____

4. A patient's husband calls the office saying his wife is having problems sleeping and is irritable. She is having nightmares about a fatal automobile accident she witnessed three months ago. She refuses to ride in a car. He is requesting an appointment. How do you handle this call?

_____

_____

_____

_____

5. A male patient calls the office and tells you he is having difficulty falling asleep and staying asleep. He also says he is physically and mentally tired, groggy, tense, irritable, and anxious in the morning. He states his sleep is not restorative. How do you handle this call?

_____

_____

_____

_____

PATIENT TEACHING

For each scenario below, outline the appropriate patient teaching you would perform. First, review the "Guidelines for Patient-Teaching Exercises" found on page iv in the "Introduction."

1. STUTTERING
   The pediatrician has seen a child after he started having episodes of stuttering. The parents have been advised that the child will probably outgrow the stuttering. The physician has printed information about many childhood communication disorders. The pediatrician suggests you provide the parents with the printed information and review it with them. How do you handle this patient (parent)-teaching opportunity?

_____

_____

_____

_____

2. DEMENTIA

The family of a patient who has recently been diagnosed with dementia caused by traumatic brain insult has made an appointment to discuss treatment and potential outcome of the insult. The physician has discussed these matters with the family. The physician has printed information regarding the potential outcome in this type of situation. She requests you review this information with the family and encourage them to ask questions in the future. How do you handle this patient (family)-teaching opportunity?

_____

_____

_____

_____

3. BIPOLAR DISORDER

A patient has just met with the physician for a review of bipolar disorder. The physician has changed the medications prescribed. He provides printed instructions and you are instructed to review this information with the patient. How do you handle this patient-teaching opportunity?

_____

_____

_____

_____

4. HYPOCHONDRIASIS

A patient has been seen numerous times for complaints with no documented basis. The physician has made a tentative diagnosis of hypochondriasis. Although the physician has printed instructions for managing these patients, she does not believe it would be in the best interest of the patient to provide him with the printed information at this time. She has reviewed the suggestions with the patient and instructs you to reinforce this information as you accompany him during the sign-out process. How will you handle this patient-teaching opportunity?

_____

_____

_____

_____

5. INSOMNIA

An individual has been experiencing periods of sleeplessness every night for the past 2 weeks. She complains of being extremely tired and of having difficulty performing routine daily activities. The physician has printed suggestions for the patient experiencing insomnia. You are instructed to provide and review these instructions with her. How do you handle this patient-teaching opportunity?

_____

_____

_____

_____

PHARMACOLOGY QUESTIONS

Circle the letter of the choice that best completes the statement or answers the question.

1. Which of the following medications are used in the treatment of ADHD?
   a. Methylphenidate (Ritalin)
   b. Amphetamine salts (Adderall)
   c. Dextroamphetamine (Dexedrine)
   d. All of the above.

2. Which of the following ADHD medications are not a DSA schedule II substance?
   a. Atomoxetine (Strattera)
   b. Methylphenidate (Ritalin)
   c. Amphetamine salts (Adderall)
   d. Dextroamphetamine (Dexedrine)

3. Which of the following medications is not a common therapy for Alzheimer's?
   a. Donepezil (Aricept)
   b. Paroxetine (Paxil)
   c. Risperidone (Risperdal)
   d. Vitamin K (Mephyton)

4. Of the following drugs of abuse, which would be considered a stimulant?
   a. Alcohol
   b. Marijuana
   c. Ketamine
   d. Cocaine

5. Many different medications have been used in the treatment of schizophrenia. Which of the following drugs could be used?
   a. Olanzapine (Zyprexa)
   b. Haloperidol (Haldol)
   c. Ziprasidone (Geodon)
   d. All of the above.

6. Depression is frequently treated with selective serotonin reuptake inhibitors (SSRIs). Which of the following is in this class?
   a. Fluoxetine (Prozac)
   b. Amitriptyline (Elavil)
   c. Nortriptyline (Pamelor)
   d. None of the above.

7. Which of the following medications could be used for the treatment of insomnia?
   a. Methylphenidate (Ritalin)
   b. Pregabalin (Lyrica)
   c. Zolpidem (Ambien)
   d. Both b & c

Essay Question

Write a response to the following question or statement. Use a separate sheet of paper if more space is needed.

Explain the physical manifestations of tic disorders. Can the person with this type of disorder control the tics?

_____

_____

_____

_____

_____

_____

_____

_____

_____

_____

_____

_____

_____

_____

_____

CERTIFICATION EXAMINATION REVIEW

Circle the letter of the choice that best completes the statement or answers the question.

1. Anxiety is a major factor that creates and maintains
   a. Autistic disorder.
   b. Mood disorder.
   c. Stuttering.
   d. All of the above.

2. Autistic disorder involves symptoms of
   a. Progressive deterioration of mental capacities.
   b. Extreme withdrawal and lack of social interaction.
   c. Anxiety resulting from an external event of an overwhelming painful nature.
   d. None of the above.

3. Haldol is the drug of choice used to treat
   a. Alzheimer's disease.
   b. Münchausen's syndrome.
   c. Tourette's disorder.
   d. None of the above.

4. Pancreatitis, cirrhosis, and peripheral neuropathy may be the result of the
   a. Prolonged, heavy use of alcohol.
   b. Occasional social drinking.
   c. Excessive use of alcohol.
   d. None of the above.

5. Bipolar disorder causes symptoms of
   a. Intense mood swings from manic to depressive.
   b. Motor tics coupled with vocal tics.
   c. Loss of concentration, fatigue, and appetite changes.
   d. All of the above.

6. The grief process has five phases. They are, in order:
   a. Anger, depression, denial, bargaining, and acceptance.
   b. Denial, anger, bargaining, depression, and acceptance.
   c. Depression, anger, denial, acceptance, and bargaining.
   d. None of the above.

7. Electroconvulsive therapy, psychotherapy, and antidepressant drug therapy may be used to treat
   a. Narcolepsy.
   b. Major depressive disorders.
   c. Somatoform disorders.
   d. All of the above.

8. Tourette's disorder is characterized by
   a. Intense mood swings from manic to depressive.
   b. Decrease in social interaction.
   c. Vocal and motor tics.
   d. None of the above.

9. Suicidal thoughts and actions may be brought on by
   a. Somatoform disorders.
   b. Autism.
   c. Major depression.
   d. None of the above.

10. Anxiety, amnesia, and impotence have been associated with
    a. Prolonged heavy use of alcohol.
    b. Excessive use of alcohol.
    c. Occasional social drinking.
    d. All of the above.

11. Panic, phobic, and obsessive-compulsive disorders are all included in the group of
    a. Somatoform disorders.
    b. Anxiety disorders.
    c. Personality disorders.
    d. None of the above.

12. Genetic disorders, infection, trauma, poisoning, early alterations in embryonic developmental general medical conditions, prematurity, or hypoxia are all identifiable causes of
    a. Autism.
    b. Mental retardation.
    c. Anxiety disorders.
    d. None of the above.

CHAPTER 15

Disorders and Conditions Resulting From Trauma

WORD DEFINITIONS

Define the following basic medical terms:

1. Amnesia _____

2. Appendage _____

3. Autograft _____

4. Axillae _____

5. Cautery _____

6. Coagulation _____

7. Constricted _____

8. Endemic _____

9. Hemostasis _____

10. Inoculation _____

11. Myalgia _____

12. Occipital _____

13. Phlebotomist _____

14. Prophylaxis _____

15. Vasculitis _____

GLOSSARY TERMS

Define the following chapter glossary terms:

1. Abduction _____

2. Anesthetic _____

3. Apnea _____

4. Cataracts _____

5. Corneal ulcers _____

6. Debrided _____

7. Electromyography (EMG) _____

8. Emergency Medical Service (EMS) _____

9. Encephalitis _____

10. Ergonomic _____

11. Maculopapular _____

12. Prothrombin time (PT) _____

13. Steri-Strips _____

14. Vectors _____

15. Venom _____

SHORT ANSWER

Answer the following questions:

1. If a patient experiences an open trauma, what type of prophylactic injection is recommended to prevent an infection?

_____

2. Intimate partner violence may also be referred to as

_____

_____

3. If a patient calls the office after being bitten by a snake, what steps should you inform them *not* to take?

_____

4. Identify the name of the rule that is used to determine the percentage of body surface area that is affected when a person sustains burn injuries.

_____

5. List some symptoms of early stage hypothermia.

_____

_____

6. Name the areas of the body that are at high risk for frostbite when exposed to extreme cold.

_____

7. Identify one disease that is transmitted by a mosquito.

_____

8. Name three diseases that may be transmitted by ticks to humans.

_____

_____

9. Name the substance that insects inject when they bite a person.

_____

10. What is the incubation time for a person to become ill between the time they are bitten by a tick and when they begin to show symptoms of Rocky Mountain spotted fever?

_____

11. Explain the best way to remove an insect stinger when it is still attached to the skin after an individual has been bitten.

_____

12. What are the mild symptoms of altitude sickness?

_____

13. List four species of poisonous snakes found in the United States.

_____

_____

14. What is one way to determine whether a poisonous snake versus a nonpoisonous snake has bitten a patient? (Disregard coral snakes.)

_____

_____

15. Identify the type of poisonous snake responsible for the greatest number of snakebites.

_____

16. Name the nerve that is entrapped when a patient has carpal tunnel syndrome.

_____

17. Are tennis players the only people who are diagnosed with tennis elbow?

_____

18. (True or false?) Deep frostbite warming should not begin until professional medical care can be provided.

_____

19. When a person experiences an electrical burn, what two things will be visible on their skin?

_____

20. Identify treatment options for carpal tunnel syndrome.

_____

_____

21. What is the health care worker's responsibility in regard to reporting suggested child abuse and neglect?

_____

_____

22. Identify the three symptoms that lead the physician to diagnose a child with shaken baby syndrome.

_____

_____

23. (True or false?) Emotional abuse is easy to identify.

_____

24. Define sexual abuse.

_____

_____

25. Name the most reliable method to determine a child's paternity.

_____

26. List examples of possible sources of danger involving bioterrorism.

_____

27. By what method could the smallpox virus be spread throughout the population?

_____

28. Identify the area of the body that would be affected if there is an outbreak of plague.

_____

FILL IN THE BLANKS

Fill in the blanks with correct terms. A word list has been provided.

1. Physical trauma is the _____ cause of death in _____ people in the United States.

2. Abrasions are caused by _____ from a _____ hard surface.

3. Puncture wounds cause _____ and very little _____.

4. The edges of a laceration may be _____ or they may be _____ depending on the object that did the cutting.

5. Anything that enters a portion of the _____ where it does not belong is considered a _____ body. Common sites for foreign bodies include the _____, the _____, the _____, and any surface area of the body.

6. Common foreign bodies in the eye include _____, _____, dust, _____, hair, small pieces of metal, small pieces of brush, or _____ branches.

7. Staining the eye with _____ to visualize a _____ abrasion will confirm the presence or previous presence of a foreign body.

8. Major burns are referred to _____ for treatment.

9. The treatment for sunburn includes cooling with cool water and spraying with _____ and _____ sprays.

10. Burns are the results of _____ insults to the tissues.

11. Patients who have experienced electrical shock may be in

    _____ or _____ failure.

12. Heat _____ occurs when the person has a body

    _____ of 105° F or higher.

13. If a person's core body temperature drops below 95° F,

    _____ will occur.

14. People with _____ _____,

    _____ _____, or scorpion bites should be

    transported to an emergency facility.

15. The antibiotic treatment of choice for Rocky Mountain spotted fever is

    _____.

WORD LIST

analgesic, antiseptic, black widow, bleeding, body, brown recluse, bugs, burn centers, cardiac, corneal, ears, eyes, fluorescin, foreign, friction, hypothermia, jagged, leading, nose, pain, respiratory, rough, rust, sand, smooth, stroke, temperature, tetracycline, thermal, tree, young

ANATOMIC STRUCTURES

Identify the following wound types.

1. _____

2. _____

3. _____

4. _____

5. _____

6. _____

PATIENT SCREENING

For each scenario below, explain how and why you would schedule an appointment or suggest a referral based on that patient's reported symptoms. First, review the "Guidelines for Patient-Screening Exercises" found on page iii in the "Introduction."

1. A father calls to report that his 4-year-old son has stepped on a nail in a board. The child pulled his foot off the board and nail, and the foot looks red around the site. He wants to know what to do. How do you handle this call?

_____

_____

_____

_____

_____

_____

2. A patient calls the office complaining of feeling a stuffiness and something in the ear. He has complaints of pain in the ear canal and decreased hearing capability. How do you respond to this call?

_____

_____

_____

_____

_____

3. A mother calls in advising her 16-year-old son has been out in the extreme cold. She has noticed the tissue on his face is firm and the skin has a waxy appearance. The skin is very cold to the touch. How do you respond to this call?

_____

_____

_____

_____

_____

4. A female patient calls in advising she is experiencing a numbness of hands and fingers with pain in these areas at night. Swelling of the wrist or hand and "fluttering" of the fingers are additional symptoms. How do you handle this call?

_____

_____

_____

_____

_____

5. An older patient calls in telling you she has noticed bruising on her daughter in various stages of healing and on areas of the body that are concealed by clothing. Her daughter says she will agree to come to the office. How do you respond?

_____

_____

_____

_____

_____

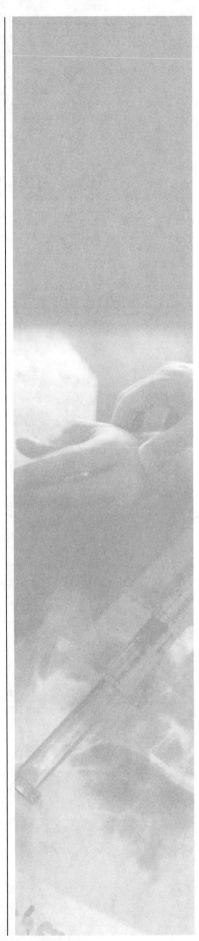

PATIENT TEACHING

For each scenario below, outline the appropriate patient teaching you would perform. First, review the "Guidelines for Patient-Teaching Exercises" found on page iv in the "Introduction."

1. AVULSION

   A patient has been involved in a traumatic situation experiencing an avulsion to the left hand. After the repair of the involved area is complete, the patient requires instruction on care of the wound. The physician has printed information regarding wound care. You are instructed to give and review this information with the patient and family. How do you handle this patient-teaching opportunity?

   _____

   _____

   _____

   _____

   _____

2. FOREIGN BODY IN THE EAR

   A parent brought their child in with a small bead in the ear canal that has been in the ear for 2 days. After the physician removed the foreign body, he discussed with the child and parent the problems that may develop when foreign bodies are in a child's ear. You are instructed to provide the parent with printed instructions regarding foreign bodies in the ears, eyes, and nose. How do you handle this patient (parent)-teaching opportunity?

   _____

   _____

   _____

   _____

   _____

3. LIGHTNING STRIKE INJURIES

   A patient was struck by lightning a few days ago. He has been released from the hospital and is in the office for a follow-up visit. Having survived the attack, the patient expresses an interest in prevention of the situation occurring again. How do you handle this patient-teaching opportunity?

   _____

   _____

   _____

   _____

   _____

4. ANIMAL BITES

A parent has brought into the office their child that has recently experienced a bite from the neighbor's dog. The child was initially treated in an emergency facility and is in the office for a follow-up examination. The parents have received patient-teaching information at the emergency facility, and a report of the incident was made to animal control. The physician requests you reinforce the printed information given to the parents by the emergency facility. How do you handle this patient-teaching opportunity?

_____

_____

_____

_____

_____

_____

5. CARPAL TUNNEL SYNDROME

A patient comes in complaining of pain to the right hand and wrist along with numbness and tingling in the arm and hand. A diagnosis of carpal tunnel syndrome is made. The physician requests you review the printed information on carpal tunnel syndrome with the patient. How do you handle this patient-teaching opportunity?

_____

_____

_____

_____

_____

_____

ESSAY QUESTION

Write a response to the following question or statement. Use a separate sheet of paper if more space is needed.

Describe the physical indicators that may be present when a child is the victim of child abuse and neglect.

_____

_____

_____

_____

_____

_____

_____

_____

_____

_____

_____

_____

_____

_____

_____

_____

_____

_____

_____

CERTIFICATION EXAMINATION REVIEW

Circle the letter of the choice that best completes the statement or answers the question.

1. Victims of abuse can include
   a. Men.
   b. Women.
   c. Children.
   d. All of the above.

2. Gentle cleansing, approximation and securing of the edges, debridement, suturing, sterile dressing application, and use of tissue glue are all methods to treat a
   a. Puncture wound.
   b. Laceration.
   c. Burn.
   d. None of the above.

3. Carpal tunnel syndrome is a repetitive motion injury that involves the _____ nerve.
   a. Sciatic
   b. Median
   c. Brachial plexus
   d. None of the above

4. An avulsion is a soft tissue injury where the
   a. Outer layer of the skin has been scraped away.
   b. Skin, tissue, and bone are being pulled away from the body.
   c. Wound has a straight neat edge.
   d. None of the above.

5. An abrasion is a soft tissue injury where the
   a. Outer layer of the skin has been scraped away.
   b. Skin, tissue, and bone are being pulled away from the body.
   c. Wound has a straight neat edge.
   d. None of the above.

6. Heat stroke causes symptoms of red, hot, dry skin; headache; dizziness; shortness of breath; and a body temperature of
   a. 102° to 104° F.
   b. 103° F.
   c. More than 105° F.
   d. None of the above.

7. Thoracic outlet syndrome involves compression of the _____ nerve.
   a. Sciatic
   b. Median
   c. Brachial plexus
   d. None of the above

8. The percentage area of the body burned is determined by using the rule of
   a. Eights.
   b. Nines.
   c. Tens.
   d. None of the above.

9. Bugs, insects, cereal, peas, beans, grapes, pebbles, and cotton are all foreign bodies sometimes found in a patient's
   a. Ears.
   b. Eyes.
   c. Eyes and ears.
   d. None of the above.

10. Treatment of frostbite includes
    a. Vigorous massage of the affected area.
    b. Immersion of the affected part in hot water.
    c. Deep rewarming supervision by health care professionals.
    d. None of the above.

11. State laws vary, but most require reporting of suggested child abuse and neglect
    a. By all people.
    b. By health care workers.
    c. By teachers.
    d. Both b and c.

12. Parentage of a child is best determined by
    a. Urinalysis.
    b. Asking the child's caregiver.
    c. DNA testing.
    d. None of the above.